THIS JOURNAL BELONGS TO:

....

....

WELLNESS IS THE COMPLETE INTEGRATION OF BODY, MIND, AND SPIRIT.

Welcome, your journey to a healthier life starts here! This comprehensive journal is a tool for you to achieve wellness. In 90 days you will grow to develop healthier habits, feel and look your best, achieve more gratitude, reach your goals and cast away unhealthy practices. Be very proud of yourself for starting this quest! You can do this!

★ ★ ★ ★ ★

Please consider supporting us by leaving a review on the retailer's website from which you acquired this journal. It helps us reach more people!
For questions or concerns email us at hello@RemoveYourShadow.com.

For a total of 90 days you will record your daily:

*Sleep goals	*Health symptoms	*Vitamins	*Food log	*Mood
*Water intake	*Self-care goals	*Gratitude	*Prompts	*Weight
*Screen time	*Supplements	*Self-care	*Fresh air & sun time	
*Affirmations	*Prayer request	*Fitness	*Personal Development	

START DATE:

(optional) Measurements

Waist: Chest:

Thighs: Hips:

Upper Arms: Calves:

Pay attention to your thoughts & overcome toxic self-criticism.
List 3 things you love about yourself.

1.

2.

3.

True joy is about letting go and changing where we seek happiness.
List 3 things you need to get rid of or work on in order to achieve more joy.

1.

2.

3.

List 3 relationships you need to work on or move on from.

1.

2.

3.

Circle how you feel today or write your own: _____

Kind   Connected   Clear   Playful   Simple   Abundant

Purposeful   Calm   Loving   Joyful   Adventurous

Open   Spiritual   Free   Faithful   Generous

What do you want to accomplish in the next 90 days (3 months)?

Sample

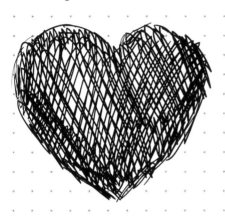

love

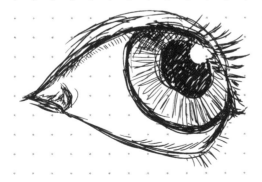

Sample

January 2022

SUNDAY	MONDAY	TUESDAY	WEDNESDAY	THURSDAY	FRIDAY	SATURDAY
						1 New Years Party!
2 Church 11:00AM	3 Homeschool Meeting 10AM	4	5	6	7	8 Bobby turns 6
9	10	11 Zumba 8AM-9AM	12	13	14	15
16	17	18 Academy 9AM-2:30PM	19	20	21	22 Date night 6PM
23	24	25	26	27 Book Club 9:30AM	28	29
30	31 Work on taxes $$$$					

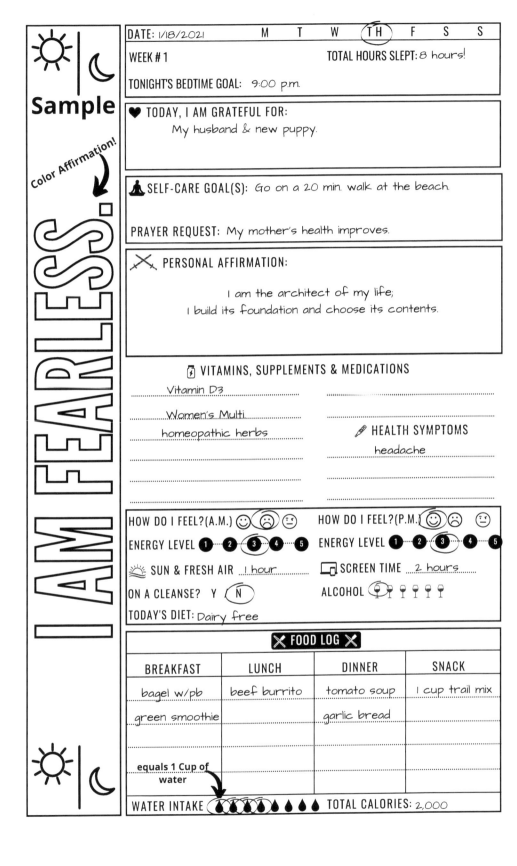

Sample

Color Affirmation!

I AM FEARLESS.

DATE: 1/18/2021   M   T   W   (TH)   F   S   S

WEEK # 1   TOTAL HOURS SLEPT: 8 hours!

TONIGHT'S BEDTIME GOAL: 9:00 p.m.

♥ TODAY, I AM GRATEFUL FOR:
> My husband & new puppy.

🧘 SELF-CARE GOAL(S): Go on a 20 min. walk at the beach.

PRAYER REQUEST: My mother's health improves.

⚔ PERSONAL AFFIRMATION:
> I am the architect of my life;
> I build its foundation and choose its contents.

⚡ VITAMINS, SUPPLEMENTS & MEDICATIONS

Vitamin D3
Women's Multi
homeopathic herbs

✎ HEALTH SYMPTOMS
headache

HOW DO I FEEL?(A.M.) ☺ ☹ 😐   HOW DO I FEEL?(P.M.) ☺ ☹ 😐

ENERGY LEVEL 1 — 2 — ③ — 4 — 5   ENERGY LEVEL 1 — 2 — ③ — 4 — 5

☀ SUN & FRESH AIR 1 hour   🖥 SCREEN TIME 2 hours

ON A CLEANSE? Y (N)   ALCOHOL 🍷 🍷 🍷 🍷 🍷

TODAY'S DIET: Dairy free

✖ FOOD LOG ✖

BREAKFAST	LUNCH	DINNER	SNACK
bagel w/pb	beef burrito	tomato soup	1 cup trail mix
green smoothie		garlic bread	
equals 1 Cup of water			

WATER INTAKE ⬗⬗⬗⬗⬗◆◆◆◆   TOTAL CALORIES: 2,000

Sample

⬤━⬤ EXERCISE LOG ⬤━⬤

(OPTIONAL) WEIGHT: 130 LBS.				START TIME	END TIME
STRETCH				10:00 a.m.	10:15 a.m.

WEIGHT TRAINING	WEIGHT	SETS	REPS	START TIME	END TIME
dumbbells	15 lbs.	4	10	10:15 a.m.	10:45 a.m.
seated high row	20 lbs.	4	10	10:45 a.m.	11:00 a.m.

CARDIO	START TIME	END TIME
100 squats	11:10 a.m.	11:25 a.m.

Circle how you feel today or write your own: ....

Kind   Connected   Clear   Playful   Simple   Abundant

Purposeful   Calm   Loving   Joyful   Adventurous

Open   Spiritual   Free   Faithful   (Generous)

What did you learn today?

It feels wonderful to be able to give to those in need.

Sample

Go to the post office & drop off package.

Buy a new lamp for my home office.

Call dance instructor before end of the week.

Create a vision board.

WELLNESS APPOINTMENTS: I hour massage at 4:00 p.m. .

NEEDS IMPROVEMENT: I need to spend more time reading and limit tv time.

INSIGHTS & LESSONS: I don't need to commit to something I don't feel comfortable with.

SUCCESSES & WINS: I finished my project on time!

◖—◗ EXERCISE LOG ◖—◗

(OPTIONAL) WEIGHT:				START TIME	END TIME
STRETCH					

WEIGHT TRAINING	WEIGHT	SETS	REPS	START TIME	END TIME

CARDIO		START TIME	END TIME

Circle how you feel today or write your own: ....

Kind	Connected	Clear	Playful	Simple	Abundant
Purposeful	Calm	Loving	Joyful		Adventurous
Open	Spiritual	Free	Faithful		Generous

What did you learn today?

I AM WORTHY

DATE:		M	T	W	TH	F	S	S

WEEK # 2   TOTAL HOURS SLEPT:

TONIGHT'S BEDTIME GOAL:

♥ TODAY, I AM GRATEFUL FOR:

🧘 SELF-CARE GOAL(S):

PRAYER REQUEST:

⚔ PERSONAL AFFIRMATION:

🔋 VITAMINS, SUPPLEMENTS & MEDICATIONS

....

....

....

....

....

🌡 HEALTH SYMPTOMS

....

....

....

HOW DO I FEEL?(A.M.) ☺ ☹ 😐   HOW DO I FEEL?(P.M.) ☺ ☹ 😐

ENERGY LEVEL ① ② ③ ④ ⑤   ENERGY LEVEL ① ② ③ ④ ⑤

🌅 SUN & FRESH AIR ....   🖥 SCREEN TIME ....

ON A CLEANSE? Y / N   ALCOHOL 🍷 🍷 🍷 🍷 🍷

TODAY'S DIET:

✗ FOOD LOG ✗

BREAKFAST	LUNCH	DINNER	SNACK

WATER INTAKE 🌢🌢🌢🌢🌢🌢🌢🌢 TOTAL CALORIES:

⬤—⬤ EXERCISE LOG ⬤—⬤

(OPTIONAL) WEIGHT:				START TIME	END TIME
STRETCH 🧘					

WEIGHT TRAINING 🏋	WEIGHT	SETS	REPS	START TIME	END TIME

CARDIO 🏃		START TIME	END TIME

Circle how you feel today or write your own: _____

Kind	Connected	Clear	Playful	Simple	Abundant
Purposeful	Calm	Loving	Joyful		Adventurous
Open	Spiritual	Free	Faithful		Generous

What did you learn today?

I AM POWERFUL

DATE:		M	T	W	TH	F	S	S

WEEK # 2   TOTAL HOURS SLEPT:

TONIGHT'S BEDTIME GOAL:

♥ TODAY, I AM GRATEFUL FOR:

🧘 SELF-CARE GOAL(S):

PRAYER REQUEST:

⚔ PERSONAL AFFIRMATION:

🔋 VITAMINS, SUPPLEMENTS & MEDICATIONS

....
....
....   🖊 HEALTH SYMPTOMS
....
....
....

HOW DO I FEEL?(A.M.) ☺ ☹ 😐   HOW DO I FEEL?(P.M.) ☺ ☹ 😐

ENERGY LEVEL ❶ ❷ ❸ ❹ ❺   ENERGY LEVEL ❶ ❷ ❸ ❹ ❺

☀ SUN & FRESH AIR ....   💻 SCREEN TIME ....

ON A CLEANSE? Y / N   ALCOHOL 🍷 🍷 🍷 🍷 🍷

TODAY'S DIET:

✗ FOOD LOG ✗

BREAKFAST	LUNCH	DINNER	SNACK

WATER INTAKE 🔴🔴🔴🔴🔴🔴🔴🔴 TOTAL CALORIES:

◁▭▷ EXERCISE LOG ◁▭▷

(OPTIONAL) WEIGHT:				START TIME	END TIME
STRETCH 🧘					

WEIGHT TRAINING 🏋	WEIGHT	SETS	REPS	START TIME	END TIME

CARDIO 🏃	START TIME	END TIME

Circle how you feel today or write your own: ....

Kind   Connected   Clear   Playful   Simple   Abundant

Purposeful   Calm   Loving   Joyful   Adventurous

Open   Spiritual   Free   Faithful   Generous

What did you learn today?

I AM THANKFUL.

DATE:	M	T	W	TH	F	S	S

WEEK # 2   TOTAL HOURS SLEPT:

TONIGHT'S BEDTIME GOAL:

♥ TODAY, I AM GRATEFUL FOR:

🧘 SELF-CARE GOAL(S):

PRAYER REQUEST:

⚔ PERSONAL AFFIRMATION:

🔋 VITAMINS, SUPPLEMENTS & MEDICATIONS

....

....

....   🌡 HEALTH SYMPTOMS

....

....

....

HOW DO I FEEL?(A.M.) ☺ ☹ 😐   HOW DO I FEEL?(P.M.) ☺ ☹ 😐

ENERGY LEVEL 1 2 3 4 5   ENERGY LEVEL 1 2 3 4 5

🌅 SUN & FRESH AIR ....   📱 SCREEN TIME ....

ON A CLEANSE? Y / N   ALCOHOL 🍷 🍷 🍷 🍷 🍷 🍷

TODAY'S DIET:

✗ FOOD LOG ✗			
BREAKFAST	LUNCH	DINNER	SNACK

WATER INTAKE 🌢🌢🌢🌢🌢🌢🌢🌢 TOTAL CALORIES:

⬤—⬤ EXERCISE LOG ⬤—⬤

(OPTIONAL) WEIGHT:				START TIME	END TIME
STRETCH					

WEIGHT TRAINING	WEIGHT	SETS	REPS	START TIME	END TIME

CARDIO		START TIME	END TIME

Circle how you feel today or write your own: ....

Kind	Connected	Clear	Playful	Simple	Abundant
Purposeful	Calm	Loving	Joyful		Adventurous
Open	Spiritual	Free	Faithful		Generous

What did you learn today?

I AM BLESSED.

DATE: M   T   W   TH   F   S   S

WEEK # 2   TOTAL HOURS SLEPT:

TONIGHT'S BEDTIME GOAL:

♥ TODAY, I AM GRATEFUL FOR:

🧘 SELF-CARE GOAL(S):

PRAYER REQUEST:

⚔ PERSONAL AFFIRMATION:

⚡ VITAMINS, SUPPLEMENTS & MEDICATIONS

....

....

....   🌡 HEALTH SYMPTOMS

....

....

....

HOW DO I FEEL?(A.M.) ☺ ☹ 😐   HOW DO I FEEL?(P.M.) ☺ ☹ 😐

ENERGY LEVEL ① ② ③ ④ ⑤   ENERGY LEVEL ① ② ③ ④ ⑤

🌅 SUN & FRESH AIR ....   💻 SCREEN TIME ....

ON A CLEANSE? Y / N   ALCOHOL 🍷 🍷 🍷 🍷 🍷

TODAY'S DIET:

⚔ FOOD LOG ⚔

BREAKFAST	LUNCH	DINNER	SNACK

WATER INTAKE 🌢🌢🌢🌢🌢🌢🌢🌢 TOTAL CALORIES:

⬤━⬤ EXERCISE LOG ⬤━⬤					

(OPTIONAL) WEIGHT:				START TIME	END TIME
STRETCH 🧘					
WEIGHT TRAINING 🏋	WEIGHT	SETS	REPS	START TIME	END TIME

CARDIO 🏃		START TIME	END TIME

Circle how you feel today or write your own: ....

Kind   Connected   Clear   Playful   Simple   Abundant

Purposeful   Calm   Loving   Joyful   Adventurous

Open   Spiritual   Free   Faithful   Generous

What did you learn today?

I AM BRAVE.

DATE: M   T   W   TH   F   S   S

WEEK # 2   TOTAL HOURS SLEPT:

TONIGHT'S BEDTIME GOAL:

❤ TODAY, I AM GRATEFUL FOR:

🧘 SELF-CARE GOAL(S):

PRAYER REQUEST:

⚔ PERSONAL AFFIRMATION:

🔋 VITAMINS, SUPPLEMENTS & MEDICATIONS

....

....

....   🌡 HEALTH SYMPTOMS

....

....

....

HOW DO I FEEL?(A.M.) ☺ ☹ 😐   HOW DO I FEEL?(P.M.) ☺ ☹ 😐

ENERGY LEVEL ❶ ❷ ❸ ❹ ❺   ENERGY LEVEL ❶ ❷ ❸ ❹ ❺

🌅 SUN & FRESH AIR ....   📱 SCREEN TIME ....

ON A CLEANSE? Y / N   ALCOHOL 🍷 🍷 🍷 🍷 🍷

TODAY'S DIET:

✖ FOOD LOG ✖

BREAKFAST	LUNCH	DINNER	SNACK

WATER INTAKE 🩸🩸🩸🩸🩸🩸🩸🩸 TOTAL CALORIES:

◀█— EXERCISE LOG —█▶

(OPTIONAL) WEIGHT:				START TIME	END TIME
STRETCH					

WEIGHT TRAINING	WEIGHT	SETS	REPS	START TIME	END TIME

CARDIO	START TIME	END TIME

Circle how you feel today or write your own: ....

| Kind | Connected | Clear | Playful | Simple | Abundant |

| Purposeful | Calm | Loving | Joyful | Adventurous |

| Open | Spiritual | Free | Faithful | Generous |

What did you learn today?

I AM CONFIDENT.

DATE: M   T   W   TH   F   S   S

WEEK # 2   TOTAL HOURS SLEPT:

TONIGHT'S BEDTIME GOAL:

♥ TODAY, I AM GRATEFUL FOR:

🧘 SELF-CARE GOAL(S):

PRAYER REQUEST:

⚔ PERSONAL AFFIRMATION:

🔋 VITAMINS, SUPPLEMENTS & MEDICATIONS

....

....

....   🌡 HEALTH SYMPTOMS

....

....

....

HOW DO I FEEL?(A.M.) ☺ ☹ 😐   HOW DO I FEEL?(P.M.) ☺ ☹ 😐

ENERGY LEVEL ❶ ❷ ❸ ❹ ❺   ENERGY LEVEL ❶ ❷ ❸ ❹ ❺

🌅 SUN & FRESH AIR ....   📺 SCREEN TIME ....

ON A CLEANSE? Y / N   ALCOHOL 🍷 🍷 🍷 🍷 🍷

TODAY'S DIET:

✗ FOOD LOG ✗

BREAKFAST	LUNCH	DINNER	SNACK

WATER INTAKE 🔴🔴🔴🔴🔴🔴🔴🔴 TOTAL CALORIES:

⊫ EXERCISE LOG ⊫

(OPTIONAL) WEIGHT:				START TIME	END TIME
STRETCH					

WEIGHT TRAINING	WEIGHT	SETS	REPS	START TIME	END TIME

CARDIO				START TIME	END TIME

Circle how you feel today or write your own: ....

| Kind | Connected | Clear | Playful | Simple | Abundant |

| Purposeful | Calm | Loving | Joyful | Adventurous |

| Open | Spiritual | Free | Faithful | Generous |

What did you learn today?

_____
_____
_____
_____
_____
_____
_____
_____
_____
_____
_____
_____
_____

WELLNESS APPOINTMENTS:
_____
_____
_____

NEEDS IMPROVEMENT:
_____
_____
_____

INSIGHTS & LESSONS:
_____
_____
_____

SUCCESSES & WINS:
_____
_____
_____

I AM FEARLESS.

DATE: M   T   W   TH   F   S   S

WEEK # 3   TOTAL HOURS SLEPT:

TONIGHT'S BEDTIME GOAL:

♥ TODAY, I AM GRATEFUL FOR:

🧘 SELF-CARE GOAL(S):

PRAYER REQUEST:

⚔ PERSONAL AFFIRMATION:

⚡ VITAMINS, SUPPLEMENTS & MEDICATIONS

....

....

....   ✏ HEALTH SYMPTOMS

....

....

HOW DO I FEEL?(A.M.) ☺ ☹ 😐   HOW DO I FEEL?(P.M.) ☺ ☹ 😐

ENERGY LEVEL ❶ ❷ ❸ ❹ ❺   ENERGY LEVEL ❶ ❷ ❸ ❹ ❺

☀ SUN & FRESH AIR ....   🖥 SCREEN TIME ....

ON A CLEANSE? Y / N   ALCOHOL 🍷 🍷 🍷 🍷 🍷

TODAY'S DIET:

✗ FOOD LOG ✗

BREAKFAST	LUNCH	DINNER	SNACK

WATER INTAKE 💧💧💧💧💧💧💧💧 TOTAL CALORIES:

⬛═⬛ EXERCISE LOG ⬛═⬛

(OPTIONAL) WEIGHT:				START TIME	END TIME
STRETCH					

WEIGHT TRAINING	WEIGHT	SETS	REPS	START TIME	END TIME

CARDIO		START TIME	END TIME

Circle how you feel today or write your own: ....

| Kind | Connected | Clear | Playful | Simple | Abundant |

| Purposeful | Calm | Loving | Joyful | Adventurous |

| Open | Spiritual | Free | Faithful | Generous |

What did you learn today?

I AM WORTHY

DATE: M   T   W   TH   F   S   S

WEEK # 3   TOTAL HOURS SLEPT:

TONIGHT'S BEDTIME GOAL:

♥ TODAY, I AM GRATEFUL FOR:

🧘 SELF-CARE GOAL(S):

PRAYER REQUEST:

⚔ PERSONAL AFFIRMATION:

⚡ VITAMINS, SUPPLEMENTS & MEDICATIONS

....

....

....   🖊 HEALTH SYMPTOMS

....

....

....

HOW DO I FEEL?(A.M.) ☺ ☹ 😐   HOW DO I FEEL?(P.M.) ☺ ☹ 😐

ENERGY LEVEL ❶ ❷ ❸ ❹ ❺   ENERGY LEVEL ❶ ❷ ❸ ❹ ❺

☀ SUN & FRESH AIR ....   🖥 SCREEN TIME ....

ON A CLEANSE? Y / N   ALCOHOL 🍷 🍷 🍷 🍷 🍷

TODAY'S DIET:

✗ FOOD LOG ✗

BREAKFAST	LUNCH	DINNER	SNACK

WATER INTAKE 🔺🔺🔺🔺🔺🔺🔺🔺 TOTAL CALORIES:

⬤▬⬤ EXERCISE LOG ⬤▬⬤

(OPTIONAL) WEIGHT:				START TIME	END TIME
STRETCH					

WEIGHT TRAINING	WEIGHT	SETS	REPS	START TIME	END TIME

CARDIO	START TIME	END TIME

Circle how you feel today or write your own: ....

Kind	Connected	Clear	Playful	Simple	Abundant
Purposeful	Calm	Loving	Joyful		Adventurous
Open	Spiritual	Free	Faithful		Generous

What did you learn today?

I AM POWERFUL.

DATE: M   T   W   TH   F   S   S

WEEK # 3   TOTAL HOURS SLEPT:

TONIGHT'S BEDTIME GOAL:

♥ TODAY, I AM GRATEFUL FOR:

🧘 SELF-CARE GOAL(S):

PRAYER REQUEST:

⚔ PERSONAL AFFIRMATION:

🔋 VITAMINS, SUPPLEMENTS & MEDICATIONS

....

....

....

....   🌡 HEALTH SYMPTOMS

....

....

HOW DO I FEEL?(A.M.) ☺ ☹ 😐   HOW DO I FEEL?(P.M.) ☺ ☹ 😐

ENERGY LEVEL ❶ ❷ ❸ ❹ ❺   ENERGY LEVEL ❶ ❷ ❸ ❹ ❺

🌅 SUN & FRESH AIR ....   📱 SCREEN TIME ....

ON A CLEANSE? Y / N   ALCOHOL 🍷 🍷 🍷 🍷 🍷

TODAY'S DIET:

✖ FOOD LOG ✖

BREAKFAST	LUNCH	DINNER	SNACK

WATER INTAKE 🔴🔴🔴🔴🔴🔴🔴🔴 TOTAL CALORIES:

⬙—⬙ EXERCISE LOG ⬙—⬙

				START TIME	END TIME
(OPTIONAL) WEIGHT:					
STRETCH					

WEIGHT TRAINING	WEIGHT	SETS	REPS	START TIME	END TIME

CARDIO		START TIME	END TIME

Circle how you feel today or write your own: ....

Kind   Connected   Clear   Playful   Simple   Abundant

Purposeful   Calm   Loving   Joyful   Adventurous

Open   Spiritual   Free   Faithful   Generous

What did you learn today?

I AM THANKFUL.

DATE: M   T   W   TH   F   S   S

WEEK # 3   TOTAL HOURS SLEPT:

TONIGHT'S BEDTIME GOAL:

♥ TODAY, I AM GRATEFUL FOR:

🧘 SELF-CARE GOAL(S):

PRAYER REQUEST:

⚔ PERSONAL AFFIRMATION:

🔋 VITAMINS, SUPPLEMENTS & MEDICATIONS

....

....

....   🌡 HEALTH SYMPTOMS

....

....

....

HOW DO I FEEL?(A.M.) ☺ ☹ 😐   HOW DO I FEEL?(P.M.) ☺ ☹ 😐

ENERGY LEVEL ❶ ❷ ❸ ❹ ❺   ENERGY LEVEL ❶ ❷ ❸ ❹ ❺

🌅 SUN & FRESH AIR ....   🖥 SCREEN TIME ....

ON A CLEANSE?   Y / N   ALCOHOL 🍷 🍷 🍷 🍷 🍷

TODAY'S DIET:

✕ FOOD LOG ✕

BREAKFAST	LUNCH	DINNER	SNACK

WATER INTAKE 🌢🌢🌢🌢🌢🌢🌢🌢 TOTAL CALORIES:

⬚➖⬚ EXERCISE LOG ⬚➖⬚

(OPTIONAL) WEIGHT:				START TIME	END TIME
STRETCH 🧘					

WEIGHT TRAINING 🏋	WEIGHT	SETS	REPS	START TIME	END TIME

CARDIO 🏃		START TIME	END TIME

Circle how you feel today or write your own: ....

Kind	Connected	Clear	Playful	Simple	Abundant

Purposeful	Calm	Loving	Joyful	Adventurous

Open	Spiritual	Free	Faithful	Generous

What did you learn today?

I AM BLESSED.

DATE: M   T   W   TH   F   S   S

WEEK # 3   TOTAL HOURS SLEPT:

TONIGHT'S BEDTIME GOAL:

♥ TODAY, I AM GRATEFUL FOR:

🧘 SELF-CARE GOAL(S):

PRAYER REQUEST:

⚔ PERSONAL AFFIRMATION:

🔋 VITAMINS, SUPPLEMENTS & MEDICATIONS

....

....

.... ✐ HEALTH SYMPTOMS

....

....

HOW DO I FEEL?(A.M.) ☺ ☹ 😐   HOW DO I FEEL?(P.M.) ☺ ☹ 😐

ENERGY LEVEL ❶ ❷ ❸ ❹ ❺   ENERGY LEVEL ❶ ❷ ❸ ❹ ❺

☀ SUN & FRESH AIR ....   🖵 SCREEN TIME ....

ON A CLEANSE? Y / N   ALCOHOL 🍷 🍷 🍷 🍷 🍷 🍷

TODAY'S DIET:

✗ FOOD LOG ✗

BREAKFAST	LUNCH	DINNER	SNACK

WATER INTAKE 🔻🔻🔻🔻🔻🔻🔻🔻 TOTAL CALORIES:

◉—◉ EXERCISE LOG ◉—◉

(OPTIONAL) WEIGHT:				START TIME	END TIME
STRETCH					

WEIGHT TRAINING	WEIGHT	SETS	REPS	START TIME	END TIME

CARDIO	START TIME	END TIME

Circle how you feel today or write your own: ....

Kind   Connected   Clear   Playful   Simple   Abundant

Purposeful   Calm   Loving   Joyful   Adventurous

Open   Spiritual   Free   Faithful   Generous

What did you learn today?

I AM BRAVE.

DATE: M   T   W   TH   F   S   S

WEEK # 3   TOTAL HOURS SLEPT:

TONIGHT'S BEDTIME GOAL:

♥ TODAY, I AM GRATEFUL FOR:

🧘 SELF-CARE GOAL(S):

PRAYER REQUEST:

✕ PERSONAL AFFIRMATION:

⚡ VITAMINS, SUPPLEMENTS & MEDICATIONS

....

....   🖊 HEALTH SYMPTOMS

....

....

....

HOW DO I FEEL?(A.M.) ☺ ☹ 😐   HOW DO I FEEL?(P.M.) ☺ ☹ 😐

ENERGY LEVEL ① ② ③ ④ ⑤   ENERGY LEVEL ① ② ③ ④ ⑤

☀ SUN & FRESH AIR ....   🖥 SCREEN TIME ....

ON A CLEANSE? Y / N   ALCOHOL 🍷 🍷 🍷 🍷 🍷

TODAY'S DIET:

✕ FOOD LOG ✕

BREAKFAST	LUNCH	DINNER	SNACK

WATER INTAKE 🔴🔴🔴🔴🔴🔴🔴🔴 TOTAL CALORIES:

⚹━━ EXERCISE LOG ━━⚹					

(OPTIONAL) WEIGHT:				START TIME	END TIME
STRETCH					

WEIGHT TRAINING	WEIGHT	SETS	REPS	START TIME	END TIME

CARDIO				START TIME	END TIME

Circle how you feel today or write your own: _____

Kind	Connected	Clear	Playful	Simple	Abundant

Purposeful	Calm	Loving	Joyful	Adventurous

Open	Spiritual	Free	Faithful	Generous

What did you learn today?

I AM CONFIDENT.

DATE: M   T   W   TH   F   S   S

WEEK # 3   TOTAL HOURS SLEPT:

TONIGHT'S BEDTIME GOAL:

♥ TODAY, I AM GRATEFUL FOR:

🧘 SELF-CARE GOAL(S):

PRAYER REQUEST:

⚔ PERSONAL AFFIRMATION:

🔋 VITAMINS, SUPPLEMENTS & MEDICATIONS

....

....

....   🖊 HEALTH SYMPTOMS

....

....

....

HOW DO I FEEL?(A.M.) ☺ ☹ 😐   HOW DO I FEEL?(P.M.) ☺ ☹ 😐

ENERGY LEVEL ❶ ❷ ❸ ❹ ❺   ENERGY LEVEL ❶ ❷ ❸ ❹ ❺

🌅 SUN & FRESH AIR ....   🖥 SCREEN TIME ....

ON A CLEANSE? Y / N   ALCOHOL 🍷 🍷 🍷 🍷 🍷

TODAY'S DIET:

✖ FOOD LOG ✖			
BREAKFAST	LUNCH	DINNER	SNACK

WATER INTAKE 🔴🔴🔴🔴🔴🔴🔴🔴 TOTAL CALORIES:

⬤—⬤ EXERCISE LOG ⬤—⬤

(OPTIONAL) WEIGHT:				START TIME	END TIME
STRETCH 🧘					

WEIGHT TRAINING 🏋	WEIGHT	SETS	REPS	START TIME	END TIME

CARDIO 🚶	START TIME	END TIME

Circle how you feel today or write your own: ....

Kind	Connected	Clear	Playful	Simple	Abundant
Purposeful	Calm	Loving	Joyful		Adventurous
Open	Spiritual	Free	Faithful		Generous

What did you learn today?

NOTES

_____

_____

_____

_____

_____

_____

_____

_____

_____

_____

_____

_____

_____

WELLNESS APPOINTMENTS:

_____

_____

_____

NEEDS IMPROVEMENT:

_____

_____

_____

INSIGHTS & LESSONS:

_____

_____

_____

SUCCESSES & WINS:

_____

_____

_____

I AM FEARLESS.

DATE: M   T   W   TH   F   S   S

WEEK # 4   TOTAL HOURS SLEPT:

TONIGHT'S BEDTIME GOAL:

♥ TODAY, I AM GRATEFUL FOR:

🧘 SELF-CARE GOAL(S):

PRAYER REQUEST:

⚔ PERSONAL AFFIRMATION:

🔋 VITAMINS, SUPPLEMENTS & MEDICATIONS

....

....

.... 🖋 HEALTH SYMPTOMS

....

....

....

HOW DO I FEEL?(A.M.) ☺ ☹ 😐   HOW DO I FEEL?(P.M.) ☺ ☹ 😐

ENERGY LEVEL ❶ ❷ ❸ ❹ ❺   ENERGY LEVEL ❶ ❷ ❸ ❹ ❺

🌅 SUN & FRESH AIR ....   🖥 SCREEN TIME ....

ON A CLEANSE? Y / N   ALCOHOL 🍷 🍷 🍷 🍷 🍷

TODAY'S DIET:

✖ FOOD LOG ✖

BREAKFAST	LUNCH	DINNER	SNACK

WATER INTAKE ♦♦♦♦♦♦♦♦♦ TOTAL CALORIES:

◖—◗ EXERCISE LOG ◖—◗					
(OPTIONAL) WEIGHT:				START TIME	END TIME
STRETCH 🧘					
WEIGHT TRAINING 🏋	WEIGHT	SETS	REPS	START TIME	END TIME
CARDIO 🏃				START TIME	END TIME

Circle how you feel today or write your own: ....

Kind	Connected	Clear	Playful	Simple	Abundant
Purposeful	Calm	Loving	Joyful		Adventurous
Open	Spiritual	Free	Faithful		Generous

What did you learn today?

I AM WORTHY.

DATE: M   T   W   TH   F   S   S

WEEK # 4   TOTAL HOURS SLEPT:

TONIGHT'S BEDTIME GOAL:

♥ TODAY, I AM GRATEFUL FOR:

🧘 SELF-CARE GOAL(S):

PRAYER REQUEST:

⚔ PERSONAL AFFIRMATION:

⚡ VITAMINS, SUPPLEMENTS & MEDICATIONS

....
....
.... ✏ HEALTH SYMPTOMS
....
....
....

HOW DO I FEEL?(A.M.) 😊 ☹ 😐   HOW DO I FEEL?(P.M.) 😊 ☹ 😐

ENERGY LEVEL ❶ ❷ ❸ ❹ ❺   ENERGY LEVEL ❶ ❷ ❸ ❹ ❺

☀ SUN & FRESH AIR ....   🖥 SCREEN TIME ....

ON A CLEANSE? Y / N   ALCOHOL 🍷 🍷 🍷 🍷 🍷

TODAY'S DIET:

⚔ FOOD LOG ⚔

BREAKFAST	LUNCH	DINNER	SNACK

WATER INTAKE 🔴🔴🔴🔴🔴🔴🔴🔴 TOTAL CALORIES:

◖▬◗ EXERCISE LOG ◖▬◗					
(OPTIONAL) WEIGHT:				START TIME	END TIME
STRETCH					
WEIGHT TRAINING	WEIGHT	SETS	REPS	START TIME	END TIME
CARDIO				START TIME	END TIME

Circle how you feel today or write your own: ....

Kind   Connected   Clear   Playful   Simple   Abundant

Purposeful   Calm   Loving   Joyful   Adventurous

Open   Spiritual   Free   Faithful   Generous

What did you learn today?

I AM POWERFUL.

DATE: M   T   W   TH   F   S   S

WEEK # 4   TOTAL HOURS SLEPT:

TONIGHT'S BEDTIME GOAL:

♥ TODAY, I AM GRATEFUL FOR:

🧘 SELF-CARE GOAL(S):

PRAYER REQUEST:

⚔ PERSONAL AFFIRMATION:

🔋 VITAMINS, SUPPLEMENTS & MEDICATIONS

....

....

....   🖊 HEALTH SYMPTOMS

....

....

....

HOW DO I FEEL?(A.M.) ☺ ☹ 😐   HOW DO I FEEL?(P.M.) ☺ ☹ 😐

ENERGY LEVEL ❶ ❷ ❸ ❹ ❺   ENERGY LEVEL ❶ ❷ ❸ ❹ ❺

☀ SUN & FRESH AIR ....   🖥 SCREEN TIME ....

ON A CLEANSE? Y / N   ALCOHOL 🍷 🍷 🍷 🍷 🍷

TODAY'S DIET:

⚔ FOOD LOG ⚔

BREAKFAST	LUNCH	DINNER	SNACK

WATER INTAKE 🔴🔴🔴🔴🔴🔴🔴🔴 TOTAL CALORIES:

⬤—⬤ EXERCISE LOG ⬤—⬤

(OPTIONAL) WEIGHT:				START TIME	END TIME
STRETCH					

WEIGHT TRAINING	WEIGHT	SETS	REPS	START TIME	END TIME

CARDIO	START TIME	END TIME

Circle how you feel today or write your own: ....

Kind	Connected	Clear	Playful	Simple	Abundant
Purposeful	Calm	Loving	Joyful		Adventurous
Open	Spiritual	Free	Faithful		Generous

What did you learn today?

I AM THANKFUL

DATE: M   T   W   TH   F   S   S

WEEK # 4   TOTAL HOURS SLEPT:

TONIGHT'S BEDTIME GOAL:

♥ TODAY, I AM GRATEFUL FOR:

🧘 SELF-CARE GOAL(S):

PRAYER REQUEST:

⚔ PERSONAL AFFIRMATION:

⚡ VITAMINS, SUPPLEMENTS & MEDICATIONS

....

....

....   🖊 HEALTH SYMPTOMS

....

....

....

HOW DO I FEEL?(A.M.) ☺ ☹ 😐   HOW DO I FEEL?(P.M.) ☺ ☹ 😐

ENERGY LEVEL ❶ ❷ ❸ ❹ ❺   ENERGY LEVEL ❶ ❷ ❸ ❹ ❺

☀ SUN & FRESH AIR ....   🖥 SCREEN TIME ....

ON A CLEANSE? Y / N   ALCOHOL 🍷 🍷 🍷 🍷 🍷

TODAY'S DIET:

✗ FOOD LOG ✗

BREAKFAST	LUNCH	DINNER	SNACK

WATER INTAKE 🌢🌢🌢🌢🌢🌢🌢🌢   TOTAL CALORIES:

EXERCISE LOG

(OPTIONAL) WEIGHT:				START TIME	END TIME
STRETCH					
WEIGHT TRAINING	WEIGHT	SETS	REPS	START TIME	END TIME
CARDIO				START TIME	END TIME

Circle how you feel today or write your own: ....

Kind Connected Clear Playful Simple Abundant

Purposeful Calm Loving Joyful Adventurous

Open Spiritual Free Faithful Generous

What did you learn today?

I AM BLESSED.

DATE:		M	T	W	TH	F	S	S

WEEK # 4   TOTAL HOURS SLEPT:

TONIGHT'S BEDTIME GOAL:

♥ TODAY, I AM GRATEFUL FOR:

🧘 SELF-CARE GOAL(S):

PRAYER REQUEST:

⚔ PERSONAL AFFIRMATION:

🔋 VITAMINS, SUPPLEMENTS & MEDICATIONS

....

....

....   🖊 HEALTH SYMPTOMS

....

....

....

HOW DO I FEEL?(A.M.) ☺ ☹ 😐   HOW DO I FEEL?(P.M.) ☺ ☹ 😐

ENERGY LEVEL ①···②···③···④···⑤   ENERGY LEVEL ①···②···③···④···⑤

🌅 SUN & FRESH AIR ....   🖥 SCREEN TIME ....

ON A CLEANSE? Y / N   ALCOHOL 🍷 🍷 🍷 🍷 🍷

TODAY'S DIET:

✖ FOOD LOG ✖

BREAKFAST	LUNCH	DINNER	SNACK

WATER INTAKE 🔴🔴🔴🔴🔴🔴🔴🔴 TOTAL CALORIES:

◖▬◗ EXERCISE LOG ◖▬◗

(OPTIONAL) WEIGHT:				START TIME	END TIME
STRETCH					

WEIGHT TRAINING	WEIGHT	SETS	REPS	START TIME	END TIME

CARDIO	START TIME	END TIME

Circle how you feel today or write your own: ....

Kind	Connected	Clear	Playful	Simple	Abundant

Purposeful	Calm	Loving	Joyful	Adventurous

Open	Spiritual	Free	Faithful	Generous

What did you learn today?

I AM BRAVE.

DATE: M   T   W   TH   F   S   S

WEEK # 4   TOTAL HOURS SLEPT:

TONIGHT'S BEDTIME GOAL:

♥ TODAY, I AM GRATEFUL FOR:

SELF-CARE GOAL(S):

PRAYER REQUEST:

PERSONAL AFFIRMATION:

🔋 VITAMINS, SUPPLEMENTS & MEDICATIONS

....

....

....   🖊 HEALTH SYMPTOMS

....

....

HOW DO I FEEL?(A.M.) ☺ ☹ 😐   HOW DO I FEEL?(P.M.) ☺ ☹ 😐

ENERGY LEVEL ❶ ❷ ❸ ❹ ❺   ENERGY LEVEL ❶ ❷ ❸ ❹ ❺

☀ SUN & FRESH AIR ....   🖥 SCREEN TIME ....

ON A CLEANSE? Y / N   ALCOHOL 🍷 🍷 🍷 🍷 🍷

TODAY'S DIET:

✕ FOOD LOG ✕			
BREAKFAST	LUNCH	DINNER	SNACK

WATER INTAKE 🌢🌢🌢🌢🌢🌢🌢🌢 TOTAL CALORIES:

⊕—⊕ EXERCISE LOG ⊕—⊕

(OPTIONAL) WEIGHT:				START TIME	END TIME
STRETCH					

WEIGHT TRAINING	WEIGHT	SETS	REPS	START TIME	END TIME

CARDIO	START TIME	END TIME

Circle how you feel today or write your own: ....

Kind   Connected   Clear   Playful   Simple   Abundant

Purposeful   Calm   Loving   Joyful   Adventurous

Open   Spiritual   Free   Faithful   Generous

What did you learn today?

I AM CONFIDENT.

DATE: M   T   W   TH   F   S   S

WEEK # 4   TOTAL HOURS SLEPT:

TONIGHT'S BEDTIME GOAL:

♥ TODAY, I AM GRATEFUL FOR:

🧘 SELF-CARE GOAL(S):

PRAYER REQUEST:

⚔ PERSONAL AFFIRMATION:

🔋 VITAMINS, SUPPLEMENTS & MEDICATIONS

....

....

....   ✏ HEALTH SYMPTOMS

....

....

....

HOW DO I FEEL?(A.M.) ☺ ☹ 😐   HOW DO I FEEL?(P.M.) ☺ ☹ 😐

ENERGY LEVEL ① ② ③ ④ ⑤   ENERGY LEVEL ① ② ③ ④ ⑤

☀ SUN & FRESH AIR ....   🖥 SCREEN TIME ....

ON A CLEANSE? Y / N   ALCOHOL 🍷 🍷 🍷 🍷 🍷

TODAY'S DIET:

✗ FOOD LOG ✗

BREAKFAST	LUNCH	DINNER	SNACK

WATER INTAKE 🔴🔴🔴🔴🔴🔴🔴🔴 TOTAL CALORIES:

⬤━⬤ EXERCISE LOG ⬤━⬤					

(OPTIONAL) WEIGHT:				START TIME	END TIME
STRETCH 🧘					

WEIGHT TRAINING 🏋	WEIGHT	SETS	REPS	START TIME	END TIME

CARDIO 🚶	START TIME	END TIME

Circle how you feel today or write your own: ....

Kind	Connected	Clear	Playful	Simple	Abundant
Purposeful	Calm	Loving	Joyful		Adventurous
Open	Spiritual	Free	Faithful		Generous

What did you learn today?

NOTES

_____

_____

_____

_____

_____

_____

_____

_____

_____

_____

_____

_____

_____

WELLNESS APPOINTMENTS:
_____

_____

_____

NEEDS IMPROVEMENT:
_____

_____

_____

INSIGHTS & LESSONS:
_____

_____

_____

SUCCESSES & WINS:
_____

_____

_____

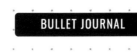

BULLET JOURNAL

SUNDAY	MONDAY	TUESDAY	WEDNESDAY	THURSDAY	FRIDAY	SATURDAY

DATE: _____ M   T   W   TH   F   S   S

WEEK # 5 _____ TOTAL HOURS SLEPT: _____

TONIGHT'S BEDTIME GOAL: _____

♥ TODAY, I AM GRATEFUL FOR:

🧘 SELF-CARE GOAL(S):

PRAYER REQUEST:

⚔ PERSONAL AFFIRMATION:

⚡ VITAMINS, SUPPLEMENTS & MEDICATIONS

....
....
....   ✏ HEALTH SYMPTOMS
....
....
....

HOW DO I FEEL?(A.M.) ☺ ☹ 😐   HOW DO I FEEL?(P.M.) ☺ ☹ 😐

ENERGY LEVEL ❶ ❷ ❸ ❹ ❺   ENERGY LEVEL ❶ ❷ ❸ ❹ ❺

🌅 SUN & FRESH AIR _____   💻 SCREEN TIME _____

ON A CLEANSE? Y / N   ALCOHOL 🍷 🍷 🍷 🍷 🍷

TODAY'S DIET: _____

⚔ FOOD LOG ⚔			
BREAKFAST	LUNCH	DINNER	SNACK

WATER INTAKE 🌢🌢🌢🌢🌢🌢🌢🌢 TOTAL CALORIES: _____

I AM FEARLESS.

⏻—⏻ EXERCISE LOG ⏻—⏻					

(OPTIONAL) WEIGHT:				START TIME	END TIME
STRETCH					

WEIGHT TRAINING	WEIGHT	SETS	REPS	START TIME	END TIME

CARDIO		START TIME	END TIME

Circle how you feel today or write your own:

Kind	Connected	Clear	Playful	Simple	Abundant
Purposeful	Calm	Loving	Joyful		Adventurous
Open	Spiritual	Free	Faithful		Generous

What did you learn today?

I AM WORTHY.

DATE: M   T   W   TH   F   S   S

WEEK # 5   TOTAL HOURS SLEPT:

TONIGHT'S BEDTIME GOAL:

♥ TODAY, I AM GRATEFUL FOR:

🧘 SELF-CARE GOAL(S):

PRAYER REQUEST:

⚔ PERSONAL AFFIRMATION:

🔋 VITAMINS, SUPPLEMENTS & MEDICATIONS

....

....   ✏ HEALTH SYMPTOMS

....

....

....

HOW DO I FEEL?(A.M.) 😊 ☹ 😐   HOW DO I FEEL?(P.M.) 😊 ☹ 😐

ENERGY LEVEL ①②③④⑤   ENERGY LEVEL ①②③④⑤

☀ SUN & FRESH AIR ....   🖥 SCREEN TIME ....

ON A CLEANSE? Y / N   ALCOHOL 🍷🍷🍷🍷🍷🍷

TODAY'S DIET:

✕ FOOD LOG ✕

BREAKFAST	LUNCH	DINNER	SNACK

WATER INTAKE 🔻🔻🔻🔻🔻🔻🔻🔻 TOTAL CALORIES:

⬤—⬤ EXERCISE LOG ⬤—⬤					
(OPTIONAL) WEIGHT:				START TIME	END TIME
STRETCH					
WEIGHT TRAINING	WEIGHT	SETS	REPS	START TIME	END TIME
CARDIO				START TIME	END TIME

Circle how you feel today or write your own: ....

Kind   Connected   Clear   Playful   Simple   Abundant

Purposeful   Calm   Loving   Joyful   Adventurous

Open   Spiritual   Free   Faithful   Generous

What did you learn today?

I AM POWERFUL.

DATE: M   T   W   TH   F   S   S

WEEK # 5   TOTAL HOURS SLEPT:

TONIGHT'S BEDTIME GOAL:

♥ TODAY, I AM GRATEFUL FOR:

🧘 SELF-CARE GOAL(S):

PRAYER REQUEST:

⚔ PERSONAL AFFIRMATION:

🔋 VITAMINS, SUPPLEMENTS & MEDICATIONS

....

....

....   🖊 HEALTH SYMPTOMS

....

....

....

HOW DO I FEEL?(A.M.) ☺ ☹ 😐   HOW DO I FEEL?(P.M.) ☺ ☹ 😐

ENERGY LEVEL ① ② ③ ④ ⑤   ENERGY LEVEL ① ② ③ ④ ⑤

🌅 SUN & FRESH AIR ....   🖥 SCREEN TIME ....

ON A CLEANSE?   Y / N   ALCOHOL 🍷 🍷 🍷 🍷 🍷

TODAY'S DIET:

✖ FOOD LOG ✖

BREAKFAST	LUNCH	DINNER	SNACK

WATER INTAKE 🌢🌢🌢🌢🌢🌢🌢🌢 TOTAL CALORIES:

⬳ EXERCISE LOG ⬳

(OPTIONAL) WEIGHT:				START TIME	END TIME
STRETCH					

WEIGHT TRAINING	WEIGHT	SETS	REPS	START TIME	END TIME

CARDIO	START TIME	END TIME

Circle how you feel today or write your own: _____

Kind   Connected   Clear   Playful   Simple   Abundant

Purposeful   Calm   Loving   Joyful   Adventurous

Open   Spiritual   Free   Faithful   Generous

What did you learn today?

I AM THANKFUL.

DATE:　　　　　　M　T　W　TH　F　S　S

WEEK # 5　　　　　　　TOTAL HOURS SLEPT:

TONIGHT'S BEDTIME GOAL:

♥ TODAY, I AM GRATEFUL FOR:

🧘 SELF-CARE GOAL(S):

PRAYER REQUEST:

⚔ PERSONAL AFFIRMATION:

⚡ VITAMINS, SUPPLEMENTS & MEDICATIONS

....　...
....　...
....　　🌡 HEALTH SYMPTOMS
....　...
....　...
....　...

HOW DO I FEEL?(A.M.) 😊 ☹ 😑　HOW DO I FEEL?(P.M.) 😊 ☹ 😑

ENERGY LEVEL ❶ ❷ ❸ ❹ ❺　ENERGY LEVEL ❶ ❷ ❸ ❹ ❺

🌅 SUN & FRESH AIR ....　🖥 SCREEN TIME ....

ON A CLEANSE?　Y / N　ALCOHOL 🍷 🍷 🍷 🍷 🍷

TODAY'S DIET:

✗ FOOD LOG ✗			
BREAKFAST	LUNCH	DINNER	SNACK

WATER INTAKE 💧💧💧💧💧💧💧💧 TOTAL CALORIES:

⬛ EXERCISE LOG ⬛

(OPTIONAL) WEIGHT:				START TIME	END TIME
STRETCH					

WEIGHT TRAINING	WEIGHT	SETS	REPS	START TIME	END TIME

CARDIO		START TIME	END TIME

Circle how you feel today or write your own: ....

| Kind | Connected | Clear | Playful | Simple | Abundant |

| Purposeful | Calm | Loving | Joyful | Adventurous |

| Open | Spiritual | Free | Faithful | Generous |

What did you learn today?

I AM BLESSED.

DATE: M   T   W   TH   F   S   S

WEEK # 5   TOTAL HOURS SLEPT:

TONIGHT'S BEDTIME GOAL:

♥ TODAY, I AM GRATEFUL FOR:

🧘 SELF-CARE GOAL(S):

PRAYER REQUEST:

⚔ PERSONAL AFFIRMATION:

🔋 VITAMINS, SUPPLEMENTS & MEDICATIONS

....
....
....
....
....

🖊 HEALTH SYMPTOMS

....
....
....

HOW DO I FEEL?(A.M.) ☺ ☹ 😐   HOW DO I FEEL?(P.M.) ☺ ☹ 😐

ENERGY LEVEL ❶ ❷ ❸ ❹ ❺   ENERGY LEVEL ❶ ❷ ❸ ❹ ❺

🌅 SUN & FRESH AIR ....   🖥 SCREEN TIME ....

ON A CLEANSE? Y / N   ALCOHOL 🍷 🍷 🍷 🍷 🍷

TODAY'S DIET:

✗ FOOD LOG ✗

BREAKFAST	LUNCH	DINNER	SNACK

WATER INTAKE 🔴🔴🔴🔴🔴🔴🔴🔴 TOTAL CALORIES:

◖▬◗ EXERCISE LOG ◖▬◗

(OPTIONAL) WEIGHT:				START TIME	END TIME
STRETCH					

WEIGHT TRAINING	WEIGHT	SETS	REPS	START TIME	END TIME

CARDIO		START TIME	END TIME

Circle how you feel today or write your own: ....

Kind   Connected   Clear   Playful   Simple   Abundant

Purposeful   Calm   Loving   Joyful   Adventurous

Open   Spiritual   Free   Faithful   Generous

What did you learn today?

I AM BRAVE.

DATE: M   T   W   TH   F   S   S

WEEK # 5   TOTAL HOURS SLEPT:

TONIGHT'S BEDTIME GOAL:

♥ TODAY, I AM GRATEFUL FOR:

🧘 SELF-CARE GOAL(S):

PRAYER REQUEST:

⚔ PERSONAL AFFIRMATION:

⚡ VITAMINS, SUPPLEMENTS & MEDICATIONS

....

....

.... ✐ HEALTH SYMPTOMS

....

....

....

HOW DO I FEEL?(A.M.) 🙂 🙁 😐   HOW DO I FEEL?(P.M.) 🙂 🙁 😐

ENERGY LEVEL ❶ ❷ ❸ ❹ ❺   ENERGY LEVEL ❶ ❷ ❸ ❹ ❺

🌅 SUN & FRESH AIR ....   🖥 SCREEN TIME ....

ON A CLEANSE? Y / N   ALCOHOL 🍷 🍷 🍷 🍷 🍷

TODAY'S DIET:

✖ FOOD LOG ✖

BREAKFAST	LUNCH	DINNER	SNACK

WATER INTAKE 🔻🔻🔻🔻🔻🔻🔻🔻 TOTAL CALORIES:

◁⊫ EXERCISE LOG ◁⊫

		START TIME	END TIME
(OPTIONAL) WEIGHT:			
STRETCH			

WEIGHT TRAINING	WEIGHT	SETS	REPS	START TIME	END TIME

CARDIO	START TIME	END TIME

Circle how you feel today or write your own: ....

Kind	Connected	Clear	Playful	Simple	Abundant
Purposeful	Calm	Loving	Joyful		Adventurous
Open	Spiritual	Free	Faithful		Generous

What did you learn today?

I AM CONFIDENT.

DATE: M   T   W   TH   F   S   S

WEEK # 5   TOTAL HOURS SLEPT:

TONIGHT'S BEDTIME GOAL:

♥ TODAY, I AM GRATEFUL FOR:

🧘 SELF-CARE GOAL(S):

PRAYER REQUEST:

⚔ PERSONAL AFFIRMATION:

⚡ VITAMINS, SUPPLEMENTS & MEDICATIONS

....

....

....   🖊 HEALTH SYMPTOMS

....

....

....

HOW DO I FEEL?(A.M.) 😊 ☹ 😐   HOW DO I FEEL?(P.M.) 😊 ☹ 😐

ENERGY LEVEL ① ② ③ ④ ⑤   ENERGY LEVEL ① ② ③ ④ ⑤

🌅 SUN & FRESH AIR ....   🖥 SCREEN TIME ....

ON A CLEANSE? Y / N   ALCOHOL 🍷 🍷 🍷 🍷 🍷

TODAY'S DIET:

✕ FOOD LOG ✕

BREAKFAST	LUNCH	DINNER	SNACK

WATER INTAKE 🔻🔻🔻🔻🔻🔻🔻🔻 TOTAL CALORIES:

⊪—⊪ EXERCISE LOG ⊪—⊪

(OPTIONAL) WEIGHT:				START TIME	END TIME
STRETCH					

WEIGHT TRAINING	WEIGHT	SETS	REPS	START TIME	END TIME

CARDIO		START TIME	END TIME

Circle how you feel today or write your own: ....

Kind	Connected	Clear	Playful	Simple	Abundant
Purposeful	Calm	Loving	Joyful		Adventurous
Open	Spiritual	Free	Faithful		Generous

What did you learn today?

_____
_____
_____
_____
_____
_____
_____
_____
_____
_____
_____
_____
_____

WELLNESS APPOINTMENTS:
_____
_____
_____

NEEDS IMPROVEMENT:
_____
_____
_____

INSIGHTS & LESSONS:
_____
_____
_____

SUCCESSES & WINS:
_____
_____
_____

I AM FEARLESS.

DATE: M   T   W   TH   F   S   S

WEEK # 6   TOTAL HOURS SLEPT:

TONIGHT'S BEDTIME GOAL:

♥ TODAY, I AM GRATEFUL FOR:

🧘 SELF-CARE GOAL(S):

PRAYER REQUEST:

⚔ PERSONAL AFFIRMATION:

⚡ VITAMINS, SUPPLEMENTS & MEDICATIONS

....

....

....   🖊 HEALTH SYMPTOMS

....

....

....

HOW DO I FEEL?(A.M.) ☺ ☹ 😐   HOW DO I FEEL?(P.M.) ☺ ☹ 😐

ENERGY LEVEL ❶ ❷ ❸ ❹ ❺   ENERGY LEVEL ❶ ❷ ❸ ❹ ❺

☀ SUN & FRESH AIR ....   🖥 SCREEN TIME ....

ON A CLEANSE? Y / N   ALCOHOL 🍷 🍷 🍷 🍷 🍷

TODAY'S DIET:

✗ FOOD LOG ✗

BREAKFAST	LUNCH	DINNER	SNACK

WATER INTAKE 🔴🔴🔴🔴🔴🔴🔴🔴 TOTAL CALORIES:

◖—◗ EXERCISE LOG ◖—◗

(OPTIONAL) WEIGHT:				START TIME	END TIME
STRETCH					

WEIGHT TRAINING	WEIGHT	SETS	REPS	START TIME	END TIME

CARDIO		START TIME	END TIME

Circle how you feel today or write your own:..

Kind	Connected	Clear	Playful	Simple	Abundant

| Purposeful | Calm | Loving | Joyful | Adventurous |

| Open | Spiritual | Free | Faithful | Generous |

What did you learn today?

I AM WORTHY

DATE: M   T   W   TH   F   S   S

WEEK # 6   TOTAL HOURS SLEPT:

TONIGHT'S BEDTIME GOAL:

♥ TODAY, I AM GRATEFUL FOR:

🧘 SELF-CARE GOAL(S):

PRAYER REQUEST:

⚔ PERSONAL AFFIRMATION:

🔋 VITAMINS, SUPPLEMENTS & MEDICATIONS

....

....

....   🌡 HEALTH SYMPTOMS

....

....

HOW DO I FEEL?(A.M.) ☺ ☹ 😐   HOW DO I FEEL?(P.M.) ☺ ☹ 😐

ENERGY LEVEL ❶ ❷ ❸ ❹ ❺   ENERGY LEVEL ❶ ❷ ❸ ❹ ❺

🌅 SUN & FRESH AIR ....   📱 SCREEN TIME ....

ON A CLEANSE? Y / N   ALCOHOL 🍷 🍷 🍷 🍷 🍷

TODAY'S DIET:

✗ FOOD LOG ✗

BREAKFAST	LUNCH	DINNER	SNACK

WATER INTAKE 🌢🌢🌢🌢🌢🌢🌢🌢 TOTAL CALORIES:

⚙—⚙ EXERCISE LOG ⚙—⚙					
(OPTIONAL) WEIGHT:				START TIME	END TIME
STRETCH 🧘					
WEIGHT TRAINING 🏋	WEIGHT	SETS	REPS	START TIME	END TIME
CARDIO 🏃				START TIME	END TIME

Circle how you feel today or write your own: ....

Kind   Connected   Clear   Playful   Simple   Abundant

Purposeful   Calm   Loving   Joyful   Adventurous

Open   Spiritual   Free   Faithful   Generous

What did you learn today?

I AM POWERFUL.

DATE: M   T   W   TH   F   S   S

WEEK # 6   TOTAL HOURS SLEPT:

TONIGHT'S BEDTIME GOAL:

♥ TODAY, I AM GRATEFUL FOR:

🧘 SELF-CARE GOAL(S):

PRAYER REQUEST:

⚔ PERSONAL AFFIRMATION:

⚡ VITAMINS, SUPPLEMENTS & MEDICATIONS

....

....

....   🖊 HEALTH SYMPTOMS

....

....

....

HOW DO I FEEL?(A.M.) ☺ ☹ 😐   HOW DO I FEEL?(P.M.) ☺ ☹ 😐

ENERGY LEVEL ❶ ❷ ❸ ❹ ❺   ENERGY LEVEL ❶ ❷ ❸ ❹ ❺

🌅 SUN & FRESH AIR ....   📱 SCREEN TIME ....

ON A CLEANSE? Y / N   ALCOHOL 🍷 🍷 🍷 🍷 🍷

TODAY'S DIET:

⚔ FOOD LOG ⚔

BREAKFAST	LUNCH	DINNER	SNACK

WATER INTAKE 🔴🔴🔴🔴🔴🔴🔴🔴 TOTAL CALORIES:

⬤—⬤ EXERCISE LOG ⬤—⬤

(OPTIONAL) WEIGHT:				START TIME	END TIME
STRETCH 🧘					

WEIGHT TRAINING 🏋️	WEIGHT	SETS	REPS	START TIME	END TIME

CARDIO 🏃		START TIME	END TIME

Circle how you feel today or write your own: ....

Kind   Connected   Clear   Playful   Simple   Abundant

Purposeful   Calm   Loving   Joyful   Adventurous

Open   Spiritual   Free   Faithful   Generous

What did you learn today?

I AM THANKFUL.

DATE: M   T   W   TH   F   S   S

WEEK # 6   TOTAL HOURS SLEPT:

TONIGHT'S BEDTIME GOAL:

♥ TODAY, I AM GRATEFUL FOR:

🧘 SELF-CARE GOAL(S):

PRAYER REQUEST:

⚔ PERSONAL AFFIRMATION:

🔋 VITAMINS, SUPPLEMENTS & MEDICATIONS

....

....

....   🖊 HEALTH SYMPTOMS

....

....

....

HOW DO I FEEL?(A.M.) 😊 😞 😐   HOW DO I FEEL?(P.M.) 😊 😞 😐

ENERGY LEVEL ❶ ❷ ❸ ❹ ❺   ENERGY LEVEL ❶ ❷ ❸ ❹ ❺

☀ SUN & FRESH AIR ....   💻 SCREEN TIME ....

ON A CLEANSE? Y / N   ALCOHOL 🍷 🍷 🍷 🍷 🍷

TODAY'S DIET:

✖ FOOD LOG ✖

BREAKFAST	LUNCH	DINNER	SNACK

WATER INTAKE 🔴🔴🔴🔴🔴🔴🔴🔴 TOTAL CALORIES:

◗━◗ EXERCISE LOG ◗━◗

(OPTIONAL) WEIGHT:				START TIME	END TIME
STRETCH					

WEIGHT TRAINING	WEIGHT	SETS	REPS	START TIME	END TIME

CARDIO	START TIME	END TIME

Circle how you feel today or write your own: _____

Kind	Connected	Clear	Playful	Simple	Abundant
Purposeful	Calm	Loving	Joyful		Adventurous
Open	Spiritual	Free	Faithful		Generous

What did you learn today?

I AM BLESSED.

DATE: M   T   W   TH   F   S   S

WEEK # 6   TOTAL HOURS SLEPT:

TONIGHT'S BEDTIME GOAL:

♥ TODAY, I AM GRATEFUL FOR:

🧘 SELF-CARE GOAL(S):

PRAYER REQUEST:

⚔ PERSONAL AFFIRMATION:

🔋 VITAMINS, SUPPLEMENTS & MEDICATIONS

....

....

....

....

....

✏ HEALTH SYMPTOMS

....

....

....

HOW DO I FEEL?(A.M.) 😊 😞 😐   HOW DO I FEEL?(P.M.) 😊 😞 😐

ENERGY LEVEL ① ② ③ ④ ⑤   ENERGY LEVEL ① ② ③ ④ ⑤

🌅 SUN & FRESH AIR ....   🖥 SCREEN TIME ....

ON A CLEANSE? Y / N   ALCOHOL 🍷 🍷 🍷 🍷 🍷

TODAY'S DIET:

✕ FOOD LOG ✕

BREAKFAST	LUNCH	DINNER	SNACK

WATER INTAKE 💧💧💧💧💧💧💧💧 TOTAL CALORIES:

⬤—⬤ EXERCISE LOG ⬤—⬤

(OPTIONAL) WEIGHT:				START TIME	END TIME
STRETCH					

WEIGHT TRAINING	WEIGHT	SETS	REPS	START TIME	END TIME

CARDIO	START TIME	END TIME

Circle how you feel today or write your own: ....

| Kind | Connected | Clear | Playful | Simple | Abundant |

| Purposeful | Calm | Loving | Joyful | Adventurous |

| Open | Spiritual | Free | Faithful | Generous |

What did you learn today?

I AM BRAVE.

DATE:	M	T	W	TH	F	S	S

WEEK # 6   TOTAL HOURS SLEPT:

TONIGHT'S BEDTIME GOAL:

♥ TODAY, I AM GRATEFUL FOR:

🧘 SELF-CARE GOAL(S):

PRAYER REQUEST:

⚔ PERSONAL AFFIRMATION:

⚡ VITAMINS, SUPPLEMENTS & MEDICATIONS

....
....
....   🖊 HEALTH SYMPTOMS
....
....
....

HOW DO I FEEL?(A.M.) ☺ ☹ 😐   HOW DO I FEEL?(P.M.) ☺ ☹ 😐

ENERGY LEVEL ❶ ❷ ❸ ❹ ❺   ENERGY LEVEL ❶ ❷ ❸ ❹ ❺

☀ SUN & FRESH AIR ....   📱 SCREEN TIME ....

ON A CLEANSE? Y / N   ALCOHOL 🍷 🍷 🍷 🍷 🍷

TODAY'S DIET:

⚔ FOOD LOG ⚔			
BREAKFAST	LUNCH	DINNER	SNACK

WATER INTAKE 🌢🌢🌢🌢🌢🌢🌢🌢 TOTAL CALORIES:

◫—◫ EXERCISE LOG ◫—◫

(OPTIONAL) WEIGHT:				START TIME	END TIME
STRETCH					

WEIGHT TRAINING	WEIGHT	SETS	REPS	START TIME	END TIME

CARDIO	START TIME	END TIME

Circle how you feel today or write your own: ....

| Kind | Connected | Clear | Playful | Simple | Abundant |

| Purposeful | Calm | Loving | Joyful | Adventurous |

| Open | Spiritual | Free | Faithful | Generous |

What did you learn today?

I AM CONFIDENT.

DATE: M   T   W   TH   F   S   S

WEEK # 6   TOTAL HOURS SLEPT:

TONIGHT'S BEDTIME GOAL:

♥ TODAY, I AM GRATEFUL FOR:

🧘 SELF-CARE GOAL(S):

PRAYER REQUEST:

⚔ PERSONAL AFFIRMATION:

⚡ VITAMINS, SUPPLEMENTS & MEDICATIONS

....

....

....   ✏ HEALTH SYMPTOMS

....

....

HOW DO I FEEL? (A.M.) ☺ ☹ 😐   HOW DO I FEEL? (P.M.) ☺ ☹ 😐

ENERGY LEVEL ❶ ❷ ❸ ❹ ❺   ENERGY LEVEL ❶ ❷ ❸ ❹ ❺

🌅 SUN & FRESH AIR ....   💻 SCREEN TIME ....

ON A CLEANSE?   Y / N   ALCOHOL 🍷 🍷 🍷 🍷 🍷

TODAY'S DIET:

✗ FOOD LOG ✗

BREAKFAST	LUNCH	DINNER	SNACK

WATER INTAKE 🔷🔷🔷🔷🔷🔷🔷🔷   TOTAL CALORIES:

◀▬▶ EXERCISE LOG ◀▬▶					

(OPTIONAL) WEIGHT:				START TIME	END TIME
STRETCH 🤸					

WEIGHT TRAINING 🏋	WEIGHT	SETS	REPS	START TIME	END TIME

CARDIO 🏃				START TIME	END TIME

Circle how you feel today or write your own: ....

Kind	Connected	Clear	Playful	Simple	Abundant
Purposeful	Calm	Loving	Joyful		Adventurous
Open	Spiritual	Free	Faithful		Generous

What did you learn today?

NOTES

_____

_____

_____

_____

_____

_____

_____

_____

_____

_____

_____

WELLNESS APPOINTMENTS:

_____

_____

NEEDS IMPROVEMENT:

_____

_____

INSIGHTS & LESSONS:

_____

_____

SUCCESSES & WINS:

_____

_____

_____

DATE: M   T   W   TH   F   S   S

WEEK # 7   TOTAL HOURS SLEPT:

TONIGHT'S BEDTIME GOAL:

♥ TODAY, I AM GRATEFUL FOR:

🧘 SELF-CARE GOAL(S):

PRAYER REQUEST:

⚔ PERSONAL AFFIRMATION:

⚡ VITAMINS, SUPPLEMENTS & MEDICATIONS

....

....

.... 🌡 HEALTH SYMPTOMS

....

....

....

HOW DO I FEEL?(A.M.) ☺ ☹ 😐   HOW DO I FEEL?(P.M.) ☺ ☹ 😐

ENERGY LEVEL ❶ ❷ ❸ ❹ ❺   ENERGY LEVEL ❶ ❷ ❸ ❹ ❺

🌅 SUN & FRESH AIR ....   📱 SCREEN TIME ....

ON A CLEANSE? Y / N   ALCOHOL 🍷 🍷 🍷 🍷 🍷

TODAY'S DIET:

✗ FOOD LOG ✗

BREAKFAST	LUNCH	DINNER	SNACK

WATER INTAKE 🔴🔴🔴🔴🔴🔴🔴🔴 TOTAL CALORIES:

I AM FEARLESS.

⬤—⬤ EXERCISE LOG ⬤—⬤

(OPTIONAL) WEIGHT:				START TIME	END TIME
STRETCH					

WEIGHT TRAINING	WEIGHT	SETS	REPS	START TIME	END TIME

CARDIO	START TIME	END TIME

Circle how you feel today or write your own: ....

Kind	Connected	Clear	Playful	Simple	Abundant

Purposeful	Calm	Loving	Joyful	Adventurous

Open	Spiritual	Free	Faithful	Generous

What did you learn today?

I AM WORTHY

DATE: M   T   W   TH   F   S   S

WEEK # 7   TOTAL HOURS SLEPT:

TONIGHT'S BEDTIME GOAL:

♥ TODAY, I AM GRATEFUL FOR:

🧘 SELF-CARE GOAL(S):

PRAYER REQUEST:

⚔ PERSONAL AFFIRMATION:

⚡ VITAMINS, SUPPLEMENTS & MEDICATIONS

....

....

🖊 HEALTH SYMPTOMS

....

....

....

HOW DO I FEEL?(A.M.) ☺ ☹ 😐   HOW DO I FEEL?(P.M.) ☺ ☹ 😐

ENERGY LEVEL ❶ ❷ ❸ ❹ ❺   ENERGY LEVEL ❶ ❷ ❸ ❹ ❺

🌅 SUN & FRESH AIR ....   📱 SCREEN TIME ....

ON A CLEANSE? Y / N   ALCOHOL 🍷 🍷 🍷 🍷 🍷

TODAY'S DIET:

⚔ FOOD LOG ⚔

BREAKFAST	LUNCH	DINNER	SNACK

WATER INTAKE 🔸🔸🔸🔸🔸🔸🔸🔸 TOTAL CALORIES:

⫶⫶ EXERCISE LOG ⫶⫶

(OPTIONAL) WEIGHT:				START TIME	END TIME
STRETCH 🧘					

WEIGHT TRAINING 🏋	WEIGHT	SETS	REPS	START TIME	END TIME

CARDIO 🏃	START TIME	END TIME

Circle how you feel today or write your own:..

Kind	Connected	Clear	Playful	Simple	Abundant
Purposeful	Calm	Loving	Joyful		Adventurous
Open	Spiritual	Free	Faithful		Generous

What did you learn today?

I AM POWERFUL.

DATE: M   T   W   TH   F   S   S

WEEK # 7   TOTAL HOURS SLEPT:

TONIGHT'S BEDTIME GOAL:

♥ TODAY, I AM GRATEFUL FOR:

🧘 SELF-CARE GOAL(S):

PRAYER REQUEST:

⚔ PERSONAL AFFIRMATION:

🔋 VITAMINS, SUPPLEMENTS & MEDICATIONS

....

....

....   🖊 HEALTH SYMPTOMS

....

....

....

HOW DO I FEEL?(A.M.) 😊 😞 😐   HOW DO I FEEL?(P.M.) 😊 😞 😐

ENERGY LEVEL ❶ ❷ ❸ ❹ ❺   ENERGY LEVEL ❶ ❷ ❸ ❹ ❺

🌅 SUN & FRESH AIR ....   📺 SCREEN TIME ....

ON A CLEANSE?   Y / N   ALCOHOL 🍷 🍷 🍷 🍷 🍷 🍷

TODAY'S DIET:

✗ FOOD LOG ✗

BREAKFAST	LUNCH	DINNER	SNACK

WATER INTAKE 🌢🌢🌢🌢🌢🌢🌢🌢 TOTAL CALORIES:

◑—◻ EXERCISE LOG ◑—◻

(OPTIONAL) WEIGHT:				START TIME	END TIME
STRETCH					

WEIGHT TRAINING	WEIGHT	SETS	REPS	START TIME	END TIME

CARDIO	START TIME	END TIME

Circle how you feel today or write your own: ....

Kind	Connected	Clear	Playful	Simple	Abundant
Purposeful	Calm	Loving	Joyful		Adventurous
Open	Spiritual	Free	Faithful		Generous

What did you learn today?

I AM THANKFUL.

DATE: M   T   W   TH   F   S   S

WEEK # 7   TOTAL HOURS SLEPT:

TONIGHT'S BEDTIME GOAL:

♥ TODAY, I AM GRATEFUL FOR:

🧘 SELF-CARE GOAL(S):

PRAYER REQUEST:

⚔ PERSONAL AFFIRMATION:

🔋 VITAMINS, SUPPLEMENTS & MEDICATIONS

....

....

.... 🖊 HEALTH SYMPTOMS

....

....

....

HOW DO I FEEL?(A.M.) ☺ ☹ 😐   HOW DO I FEEL?(P.M.) ☺ ☹ 😐

ENERGY LEVEL ❶ ❷ ❸ ❹ ❺   ENERGY LEVEL ❶ ❷ ❸ ❹ ❺

☀ SUN & FRESH AIR ....   🖥 SCREEN TIME ....

ON A CLEANSE?   Y / N   ALCOHOL 🍷 🍷 🍷 🍷 🍷 🍷

TODAY'S DIET:

✕ FOOD LOG ✕

BREAKFAST	LUNCH	DINNER	SNACK

WATER INTAKE 💧💧💧💧💧💧💧💧 TOTAL CALORIES:

◑—◐ EXERCISE LOG ◑—◐

(OPTIONAL) WEIGHT:				START TIME	END TIME
STRETCH					

WEIGHT TRAINING	WEIGHT	SETS	REPS	START TIME	END TIME

CARDIO				START TIME	END TIME

Circle how you feel today or write your own: ....

Kind	Connected	Clear	Playful	Simple	Abundant
Purposeful	Calm	Loving	Joyful		Adventurous
Open	Spiritual	Free	Faithful		Generous

What did you learn today?

I AM BLESSED.

DATE: M   T   W   TH   F   S   S

WEEK # 7   TOTAL HOURS SLEPT:

TONIGHT'S BEDTIME GOAL:

♥ TODAY, I AM GRATEFUL FOR:

🧘 SELF-CARE GOAL(S):

PRAYER REQUEST:

⚔ PERSONAL AFFIRMATION:

🔋 VITAMINS, SUPPLEMENTS & MEDICATIONS

....
....
.... 🔖 HEALTH SYMPTOMS
....
....
....

HOW DO I FEEL?(A.M.) ☺ ☹ 😐   HOW DO I FEEL?(P.M.) ☺ ☹ 😐

ENERGY LEVEL ❶ ❷ ❸ ❹ ❺   ENERGY LEVEL ❶ ❷ ❸ ❹ ❺

☀ SUN & FRESH AIR ....   🖥 SCREEN TIME ....

ON A CLEANSE? Y / N   ALCOHOL 🍷 🍷 🍷 🍷 🍷

TODAY'S DIET:

✖ FOOD LOG ✖

BREAKFAST	LUNCH	DINNER	SNACK

WATER INTAKE 🔴🔴🔴🔴🔴🔴🔴🔴 TOTAL CALORIES:

◖—◗ EXERCISE LOG ◖—◗

				START TIME	END TIME
(OPTIONAL) WEIGHT:					
STRETCH 🤸					

WEIGHT TRAINING 🏋	WEIGHT	SETS	REPS	START TIME	END TIME

CARDIO 🏃	START TIME	END TIME

Circle how you feel today or write your own: ....

Kind	Connected	Clear	Playful	Simple	Abundant
Purposeful	Calm	Loving	Joyful		Adventurous
Open	Spiritual	Free	Faithful		Generous

What did you learn today?

I AM BRAVE.

DATE: M   T   W   TH   F   S   S

WEEK # 7   TOTAL HOURS SLEPT:

TONIGHT'S BEDTIME GOAL:

♥ TODAY, I AM GRATEFUL FOR:

🧘 SELF-CARE GOAL(S):

PRAYER REQUEST:

⚔ PERSONAL AFFIRMATION:

🔋 VITAMINS, SUPPLEMENTS & MEDICATIONS

....
....
....
....
....

🌡 HEALTH SYMPTOMS

HOW DO I FEEL?(A.M.) ☺ ☹ 😐   HOW DO I FEEL?(P.M.) ☺ ☹ 😐

ENERGY LEVEL ❶ ❷ ❸ ❹ ❺   ENERGY LEVEL ❶ ❷ ❸ ❹ ❺

🌅 SUN & FRESH AIR ....   🖥 SCREEN TIME ....

ON A CLEANSE? Y / N   ALCOHOL 🍷 🍷 🍷 🍷 🍷

TODAY'S DIET:

✗ FOOD LOG ✗

BREAKFAST	LUNCH	DINNER	SNACK

WATER INTAKE 🔴🔴🔴🔴🔴🔴🔴🔴 TOTAL CALORIES:

◁—▷ EXERCISE LOG ◁—▷

(OPTIONAL) WEIGHT:				START TIME	END TIME
STRETCH					

WEIGHT TRAINING	WEIGHT	SETS	REPS	START TIME	END TIME

CARDIO	START TIME	END TIME

Circle how you feel today or write your own: ....

Kind	Connected	Clear	Playful	Simple	Abundant

Purposeful   Calm   Loving   Joyful   Adventurous

Open   Spiritual   Free   Faithful   Generous

What did you learn today?

I AM CONFIDENT.

DATE: M   T   W   TH   F   S   S

WEEK # 7   TOTAL HOURS SLEPT:

TONIGHT'S BEDTIME GOAL:

♥ TODAY, I AM GRATEFUL FOR:

🧘 SELF-CARE GOAL(S):

PRAYER REQUEST:

⚔ PERSONAL AFFIRMATION:

💊 VITAMINS, SUPPLEMENTS & MEDICATIONS

....

....

.... 🌡 HEALTH SYMPTOMS

....

....

....

HOW DO I FEEL?(A.M.) ☺ ☹ 😐   HOW DO I FEEL?(P.M.) ☺ ☹ 😐

ENERGY LEVEL ❶ ❷ ❸ ❹ ❺   ENERGY LEVEL ❶ ❷ ❸ ❹ ❺

🌅 SUN & FRESH AIR ....   📺 SCREEN TIME ....

ON A CLEANSE?   Y / N   ALCOHOL 🍷 🍷 🍷 🍷 🍷

TODAY'S DIET:

✖ FOOD LOG ✖

BREAKFAST	LUNCH	DINNER	SNACK

WATER INTAKE 🔻🔻🔻🔻🔻🔻🔻🔻 TOTAL CALORIES:

⬱—◻ EXERCISE LOG ◻—⬱

(OPTIONAL) WEIGHT:				START TIME	END TIME
STRETCH 🧘					

WEIGHT TRAINING 🏋	WEIGHT	SETS	REPS	START TIME	END TIME

CARDIO 🚶	START TIME	END TIME

Circle how you feel today or write your own: ....

Kind	Connected	Clear	Playful	Simple	Abundant
Purposeful	Calm	Loving	Joyful		Adventurous
Open	Spiritual	Free	Faithful		Generous

What did you learn today?

NOTES

_____

_____

_____

_____

_____

_____

_____

_____

_____

_____

_____

_____

WELLNESS APPOINTMENTS:

_____

_____

NEEDS IMPROVEMENT:

_____

_____

INSIGHTS & LESSONS:

_____

_____

SUCCESSES & WINS:

_____

_____

_____

I AM FEARLESS.

DATE: M   T   W   TH   F   S   S

WEEK # 8   TOTAL HOURS SLEPT:

TONIGHT'S BEDTIME GOAL:

♥ TODAY, I AM GRATEFUL FOR:

🧘 SELF-CARE GOAL(S):

PRAYER REQUEST:

⚔ PERSONAL AFFIRMATION:

🔋 VITAMINS, SUPPLEMENTS & MEDICATIONS

....

.... 🌡 HEALTH SYMPTOMS

....

....

....

....

HOW DO I FEEL?(A.M.) ☺ ☹ 😐   HOW DO I FEEL?(P.M.) ☺ ☹ 😐

ENERGY LEVEL ❶ ❷ ❸ ❹ ❺   ENERGY LEVEL ❶ ❷ ❸ ❹ ❺

🌅 SUN & FRESH AIR ....   📺 SCREEN TIME ....

ON A CLEANSE? Y / N   ALCOHOL 🍷 🍷 🍷 🍷 🍷

TODAY'S DIET:

✖ FOOD LOG ✖

BREAKFAST	LUNCH	DINNER	SNACK

WATER INTAKE 🌢🌢🌢🌢🌢🌢🌢🌢 TOTAL CALORIES:

⬤—⬤ EXERCISE LOG ⬤—⬤

(OPTIONAL) WEIGHT:				START TIME	END TIME
STRETCH					

WEIGHT TRAINING	WEIGHT	SETS	REPS	START TIME	END TIME

CARDIO		START TIME	END TIME

Circle how you feel today or write your own: ....

Kind	Connected	Clear	Playful	Simple	Abundant
Purposeful	Calm	Loving	Joyful		Adventurous
Open	Spiritual	Free	Faithful		Generous

What did you learn today?

DATE: M   T   W   TH   F   S   S

WEEK # 8   TOTAL HOURS SLEPT:

TONIGHT'S BEDTIME GOAL:

♥ TODAY, I AM GRATEFUL FOR:

🧘 SELF-CARE GOAL(S):

PRAYER REQUEST:

⚔ PERSONAL AFFIRMATION:

🔋 VITAMINS, SUPPLEMENTS & MEDICATIONS

....

....   🖊 HEALTH SYMPTOMS

....

....

....

HOW DO I FEEL?(A.M.) ☺ ☹ 😐   HOW DO I FEEL?(P.M.) ☺ ☹ 😐

ENERGY LEVEL ❶ ❷ ❸ ❹ ❺   ENERGY LEVEL ❶ ❷ ❸ ❹ ❺

☀ SUN & FRESH AIR ....   🖥 SCREEN TIME ....

ON A CLEANSE?   Y / N   ALCOHOL 🍷 🍷 🍷 🍷 🍷

TODAY'S DIET:

✗ FOOD LOG ✗

BREAKFAST	LUNCH	DINNER	SNACK

WATER INTAKE 🔻🔻🔻🔻🔻🔻🔻🔻 TOTAL CALORIES:

I AM WORTHY.

◐—◑ EXERCISE LOG ◐—◑

(OPTIONAL) WEIGHT:				START TIME	END TIME
STRETCH 🧘					

WEIGHT TRAINING 🏋	WEIGHT	SETS	REPS	START TIME	END TIME

CARDIO 🏃				START TIME	END TIME

Circle how you feel today or write your own: ....

Kind	Connected	Clear	Playful	Simple	Abundant
Purposeful	Calm	Loving	Joyful		Adventurous
Open	Spiritual	Free	Faithful		Generous

What did you learn today?

I AM POWERFUL.

DATE:		M	T	W	TH	F	S	S

WEEK # 8   TOTAL HOURS SLEPT:

TONIGHT'S BEDTIME GOAL:

♥ TODAY, I AM GRATEFUL FOR:

🧘 SELF-CARE GOAL(S):

PRAYER REQUEST:

⚔ PERSONAL AFFIRMATION:

⚡ VITAMINS, SUPPLEMENTS & MEDICATIONS

....
....
....   🖊 HEALTH SYMPTOMS
....
....
....

HOW DO I FEEL?(A.M.) ☺ ☹ 😐   HOW DO I FEEL?(P.M.) ☺ ☹ 😐

ENERGY LEVEL ❶ ❷ ❸ ❹ ❺   ENERGY LEVEL ❶ ❷ ❸ ❹ ❺

🌅 SUN & FRESH AIR ....   🖥 SCREEN TIME ....

ON A CLEANSE? Y / N   ALCOHOL 🍷 🍷 🍷 🍷 🍷 🍷

TODAY'S DIET:

✕ FOOD LOG ✕			
BREAKFAST	LUNCH	DINNER	SNACK

WATER INTAKE 🟊🟊🟊🟊🟊🟊🟊🟊 TOTAL CALORIES:

◁—▷ EXERCISE LOG ◁—▷

(OPTIONAL) WEIGHT:				START TIME	END TIME
STRETCH 🧘					

WEIGHT TRAINING 🏋	WEIGHT	SETS	REPS	START TIME	END TIME

CARDIO 🏃	START TIME	END TIME

Circle how you feel today or write your own: ....

Kind	Connected	Clear	Playful	Simple	Abundant
Purposeful	Calm	Loving	Joyful		Adventurous
Open	Spiritual	Free	Faithful		Generous

What did you learn today?

I AM THANKFUL

DATE:	M T W TH F S S
WEEK # 8	TOTAL HOURS SLEPT:
TONIGHT'S BEDTIME GOAL:	

♥ TODAY, I AM GRATEFUL FOR:

🧘 SELF-CARE GOAL(S):

PRAYER REQUEST:

⚔ PERSONAL AFFIRMATION:

🔋 VITAMINS, SUPPLEMENTS & MEDICATIONS

....
....
....
....
....

✏ HEALTH SYMPTOMS

....
....
....

HOW DO I FEEL?(A.M.) ☺ ☹ 😐   HOW DO I FEEL?(P.M.) ☺ ☹ 😐

ENERGY LEVEL ① ② ③ ④ ⑤   ENERGY LEVEL ① ② ③ ④ ⑤

☀ SUN & FRESH AIR ....   💻 SCREEN TIME ....

ON A CLEANSE? Y / N   ALCOHOL 🍷 🍷 🍷 🍷 🍷

TODAY'S DIET:

✖ FOOD LOG ✖

BREAKFAST	LUNCH	DINNER	SNACK

WATER INTAKE 💧💧💧💧💧💧💧💧 TOTAL CALORIES:

◀▬▶ EXERCISE LOG ◀▬▶

(OPTIONAL) WEIGHT:				START TIME	END TIME
STRETCH					

WEIGHT TRAINING	WEIGHT	SETS	REPS	START TIME	END TIME

CARDIO	START TIME	END TIME

Circle how you feel today or write your own: ....

Kind   Connected   Clear   Playful   Simple   Abundant

Purposeful   Calm   Loving   Joyful   Adventurous

Open   Spiritual   Free   Faithful   Generous

What did you learn today?

I AM BLESSED.

DATE: M   T   W   TH   F   S   S

WEEK # 8   TOTAL HOURS SLEPT:

TONIGHT'S BEDTIME GOAL:

♥ TODAY, I AM GRATEFUL FOR:

🧘 SELF-CARE GOAL(S):

PRAYER REQUEST:

⚔ PERSONAL AFFIRMATION:

🔋 VITAMINS, SUPPLEMENTS & MEDICATIONS

....

....

....   🖋 HEALTH SYMPTOMS

....

....

....

HOW DO I FEEL?(A.M.) ☺ ☹ 😕   HOW DO I FEEL?(P.M.) ☺ ☹ 😕

ENERGY LEVEL ➊ ➋ ➌ ➍ ➎   ENERGY LEVEL ➊ ➋ ➌ ➍ ➎

🌅 SUN & FRESH AIR ....   🖥 SCREEN TIME ....

ON A CLEANSE?   Y / N   ALCOHOL 🍷 🍷 🍷 🍷 🍷

TODAY'S DIET:

⚔ FOOD LOG ⚔			
BREAKFAST	LUNCH	DINNER	SNACK

WATER INTAKE 🌑🌑🌑🌑🌑🌑🌑🌑   TOTAL CALORIES:

⬧—⬧ EXERCISE LOG ⬧—⬧

(OPTIONAL) WEIGHT:				START TIME	END TIME
STRETCH 🧘					

WEIGHT TRAINING 🏋	WEIGHT	SETS	REPS	START TIME	END TIME

CARDIO 🏃	START TIME	END TIME

Circle how you feel today or write your own:...

Kind   Connected   Clear   Playful   Simple   Abundant

Purposeful   Calm   Loving   Joyful   Adventurous

Open   Spiritual   Free   Faithful   Generous

What did you learn today?

I AM BRAVE.

DATE: M   T   W   TH   F   S   S

WEEK # 8   TOTAL HOURS SLEPT:

TONIGHT'S BEDTIME GOAL:

♥ TODAY, I AM GRATEFUL FOR:

🧘 SELF-CARE GOAL(S):

PRAYER REQUEST:

⚔ PERSONAL AFFIRMATION:

🔋 VITAMINS, SUPPLEMENTS & MEDICATIONS

....

....

....   🖊 HEALTH SYMPTOMS

....

....

....

HOW DO I FEEL?(A.M.) ☺ ☹ 😐   HOW DO I FEEL?(P.M.) ☺ ☹ 😐

ENERGY LEVEL ❶ ❷ ❸ ❹ ❺   ENERGY LEVEL ❶ ❷ ❸ ❹ ❺

☀ SUN & FRESH AIR ....   🖥 SCREEN TIME ....

ON A CLEANSE?   Y / N   ALCOHOL 🍷 🍷 🍷 🍷 🍷

TODAY'S DIET:

✗ FOOD LOG ✗

BREAKFAST	LUNCH	DINNER	SNACK

WATER INTAKE 🟤🟤🟤🟤🟤🟤🟤🟤 TOTAL CALORIES:

◧—◧ EXERCISE LOG ◧—◧

(OPTIONAL) WEIGHT:				START TIME	END TIME
STRETCH					

WEIGHT TRAINING	WEIGHT	SETS	REPS	START TIME	END TIME

CARDIO	START TIME	END TIME

Circle how you feel today or write your own: ....

Kind   Connected   Clear   Playful   Simple   Abundant

Purposeful   Calm   Loving   Joyful   Adventurous

Open   Spiritual   Free   Faithful   Generous

What did you learn today?

I AM CONFIDENT.

DATE: M   T   W   TH   F   S   S

WEEK # 8   TOTAL HOURS SLEPT:

TONIGHT'S BEDTIME GOAL:

♥ TODAY, I AM GRATEFUL FOR:

🧘 SELF-CARE GOAL(S):

PRAYER REQUEST:

⚔ PERSONAL AFFIRMATION:

🔋 VITAMINS, SUPPLEMENTS & MEDICATIONS

....

....

....   🌡 HEALTH SYMPTOMS

....

....

....

HOW DO I FEEL?(A.M.) ☺ ☹ 😐   HOW DO I FEEL?(P.M.) ☺ ☹ 😐

ENERGY LEVEL ❶ ❷ ❸ ❹ ❺   ENERGY LEVEL ❶ ❷ ❸ ❹ ❺

🌅 SUN & FRESH AIR ....   🖥 SCREEN TIME ....

ON A CLEANSE? Y / N   ALCOHOL 🍷 🍷 🍷 🍷 🍷

TODAY'S DIET:

✖ FOOD LOG ✖

BREAKFAST	LUNCH	DINNER	SNACK

WATER INTAKE 💧💧💧💧💧💧💧💧 TOTAL CALORIES:

◀—▮ EXERCISE LOG ▮—▶					

(OPTIONAL) WEIGHT:				START TIME	END TIME
STRETCH 🧘					
WEIGHT TRAINING 🏋	WEIGHT	SETS	REPS	START TIME	END TIME
CARDIO 🏃				START TIME	END TIME

Circle how you feel today or write your own: ....

Kind	Connected	Clear	Playful	Simple	Abundant
Purposeful	Calm	Loving	Joyful		Adventurous
Open	Spiritual	Free	Faithful		Generous

What did you learn today?

_____

_____

_____

_____

_____

_____

_____

_____

_____

_____

_____

_____

_____

_____

WELLNESS APPOINTMENTS:

_____

_____

NEEDS IMPROVEMENT:

_____

_____

INSIGHTS & LESSONS:

_____

_____

SUCCESSES & WINS:

_____

_____

_____

SUNDAY	MONDAY	TUESDAY	WEDNESDAY	THURSDAY	FRIDAY	SATURDAY

I AM FEARLESS.

DATE:		M	T	W	TH	F	S	S

WEEK # 9   TOTAL HOURS SLEPT:

TONIGHT'S BEDTIME GOAL:

♥ TODAY, I AM GRATEFUL FOR:

🧘 SELF-CARE GOAL(S):

PRAYER REQUEST:

⚔ PERSONAL AFFIRMATION:

🔋 VITAMINS, SUPPLEMENTS & MEDICATIONS

....

....

....   ✏ HEALTH SYMPTOMS

....

....

....

HOW DO I FEEL?(A.M.) ☺ ☹ 😐   HOW DO I FEEL?(P.M.) ☺ ☹ 😐

ENERGY LEVEL ❶ ❷ ❸ ❹ ❺   ENERGY LEVEL ❶ ❷ ❸ ❹ ❺

☀ SUN & FRESH AIR ....   🖥 SCREEN TIME ....

ON A CLEANSE? Y / N   ALCOHOL 🍷 🍷 🍷 🍷 🍷

TODAY'S DIET:

✗ FOOD LOG ✗

BREAKFAST	LUNCH	DINNER	SNACK

WATER INTAKE 🌢🌢🌢🌢🌢🌢🌢🌢 TOTAL CALORIES:

◁—▷ EXERCISE LOG ◁—▷

(OPTIONAL) WEIGHT:				START TIME	END TIME
STRETCH 🧘					

WEIGHT TRAINING 🏋	WEIGHT	SETS	REPS	START TIME	END TIME

CARDIO 🏃	START TIME	END TIME

Circle how you feel today or write your own: ....

Kind	Connected	Clear	Playful	Simple	Abundant
Purposeful	Calm	Loving	Joyful		Adventurous
Open	Spiritual	Free	Faithful		Generous

What did you learn today?

DATE: M   T   W   TH   F   S   S

WEEK # 9   TOTAL HOURS SLEPT:

TONIGHT'S BEDTIME GOAL:

♥ TODAY, I AM GRATEFUL FOR:

🧘 SELF-CARE GOAL(S):

PRAYER REQUEST:

⚔ PERSONAL AFFIRMATION:

⚡ VITAMINS, SUPPLEMENTS & MEDICATIONS

....

....   🖊 HEALTH SYMPTOMS

....

....

....

HOW DO I FEEL?(A.M.) 🙂 ☹ 😐   HOW DO I FEEL?(P.M.) 🙂 ☹ 😐

ENERGY LEVEL ❶ ❷ ❸ ❹ ❺   ENERGY LEVEL ❶ ❷ ❸ ❹ ❺

🌅 SUN & FRESH AIR ....   📱 SCREEN TIME ....

ON A CLEANSE? Y / N   ALCOHOL 🍷 🍷 🍷 🍷 🍷

TODAY'S DIET:

✗ FOOD LOG ✗

BREAKFAST	LUNCH	DINNER	SNACK

WATER INTAKE 🔻🔻🔻🔻🔻🔻🔻🔻 TOTAL CALORIES:

I AM WORTHY.

⬤—⬤ EXERCISE LOG ⬤—⬤

(OPTIONAL) WEIGHT:				START TIME	END TIME
STRETCH					
WEIGHT TRAINING	WEIGHT	SETS	REPS	START TIME	END TIME

CARDIO	START TIME	END TIME

Circle how you feel today or write your own: ....

Kind	Connected	Clear	Playful	Simple	Abundant
Purposeful	Calm	Loving	Joyful		Adventurous
Open	Spiritual	Free	Faithful		Generous

What did you learn today?

I AM POWERFUL.

DATE:		M	T	W	TH	F	S	S

WEEK # 9   TOTAL HOURS SLEPT:

TONIGHT'S BEDTIME GOAL:

♥ TODAY, I AM GRATEFUL FOR:

🧘 SELF-CARE GOAL(S):

PRAYER REQUEST:

⚔ PERSONAL AFFIRMATION:

🔋 VITAMINS, SUPPLEMENTS & MEDICATIONS

....

....

....   🌡 HEALTH SYMPTOMS

....

....

....

....

HOW DO I FEEL?(A.M.) ☺ ☹ 😐   HOW DO I FEEL?(P.M.) ☺ ☹ 😐

ENERGY LEVEL ❶ ❷ ❸ ❹ ❺   ENERGY LEVEL ❶ ❷ ❸ ❹ ❺

🌅 SUN & FRESH AIR ....   📱 SCREEN TIME ....

ON A CLEANSE? Y / N   ALCOHOL 🍷 🍷 🍷 🍷 🍷

TODAY'S DIET:

✖ FOOD LOG ✖

BREAKFAST	LUNCH	DINNER	SNACK

WATER INTAKE 🔹🔹🔹🔹🔹🔹🔹🔹 TOTAL CALORIES:

◖—◗ EXERCISE LOG ◖—◗

(OPTIONAL) WEIGHT:				START TIME	END TIME
STRETCH					

WEIGHT TRAINING	WEIGHT	SETS	REPS	START TIME	END TIME

CARDIO	START TIME	END TIME

Circle how you feel today or write your own: ....

Kind   Connected   Clear   Playful   Simple   Abundant

Purposeful   Calm   Loving   Joyful   Adventurous

Open   Spiritual   Free   Faithful   Generous

What did you learn today?

I AM THANKFUL.

DATE: M   T   W   TH   F   S   S

WEEK # 9   TOTAL HOURS SLEPT:

TONIGHT'S BEDTIME GOAL:

♥ TODAY, I AM GRATEFUL FOR:

🧘 SELF-CARE GOAL(S):

PRAYER REQUEST:

⚔ PERSONAL AFFIRMATION:

🔋 VITAMINS, SUPPLEMENTS & MEDICATIONS

....

....

.... 🖊 HEALTH SYMPTOMS

....

....

....

HOW DO I FEEL?(A.M.) ☺ ☹ 😐   HOW DO I FEEL?(P.M.) ☺ ☹ 😐

ENERGY LEVEL ① ② ③ ④ ⑤   ENERGY LEVEL ① ② ③ ④ ⑤

☀ SUN & FRESH AIR ....   📱 SCREEN TIME ....

ON A CLEANSE? Y / N   ALCOHOL 🍷 🍷 🍷 🍷 🍷 🍷

TODAY'S DIET:

✕ FOOD LOG ✕

BREAKFAST	LUNCH	DINNER	SNACK

WATER INTAKE 🌢🌢🌢🌢🌢🌢🌢🌢 TOTAL CALORIES:

◖—◗ EXERCISE LOG ◖—◗

(OPTIONAL) WEIGHT:				START TIME	END TIME
STRETCH					
WEIGHT TRAINING	WEIGHT	SETS	REPS	START TIME	END TIME

CARDIO		START TIME	END TIME

Circle how you feel today or write your own: ....

Kind	Connected	Clear	Playful	Simple	Abundant
Purposeful	Calm	Loving	Joyful		Adventurous
Open	Spiritual	Free	Faithful		Generous

What did you learn today?

I AM BLESSED.

DATE: M   T   W   TH   F   S   S

WEEK # 9   TOTAL HOURS SLEPT:

TONIGHT'S BEDTIME GOAL:

♥ TODAY, I AM GRATEFUL FOR:

🧘 SELF-CARE GOAL(S):

PRAYER REQUEST:

⚔ PERSONAL AFFIRMATION:

🔋 VITAMINS, SUPPLEMENTS & MEDICATIONS

....

....

....   ✏ HEALTH SYMPTOMS

....

....

....

HOW DO I FEEL?(A.M.) ☺ ☹ 😐   HOW DO I FEEL?(P.M.) ☺ ☹ 😐

ENERGY LEVEL ❶ ❷ ❸ ❹ ❺   ENERGY LEVEL ❶ ❷ ❸ ❹ ❺

☀ SUN & FRESH AIR ....   🖥 SCREEN TIME ....

ON A CLEANSE? Y / N   ALCOHOL 🍷 🍷 🍷 🍷 🍷

TODAY'S DIET:

✖ FOOD LOG ✖			
BREAKFAST	LUNCH	DINNER	SNACK

WATER INTAKE 💧💧💧💧💧💧💧💧 TOTAL CALORIES:

◁▤▷ EXERCISE LOG ◁▤▷

(OPTIONAL) WEIGHT:				START TIME	END TIME
STRETCH					
WEIGHT TRAINING	WEIGHT	SETS	REPS	START TIME	END TIME

CARDIO		START TIME	END TIME

Circle how you feel today or write your own: ....

Kind	Connected	Clear	Playful	Simple	Abundant
Purposeful	Calm	Loving	Joyful		Adventurous
Open	Spiritual	Free	Faithful		Generous

What did you learn today?

I AM BRAVE.

DATE: M   T   W   TH   F   S   S

WEEK # 9   TOTAL HOURS SLEPT:

TONIGHT'S BEDTIME GOAL:

♥ TODAY, I AM GRATEFUL FOR:

🧘 SELF-CARE GOAL(S):

PRAYER REQUEST:

⚔ PERSONAL AFFIRMATION:

🔋 VITAMINS, SUPPLEMENTS & MEDICATIONS

....

....

....   🖊 HEALTH SYMPTOMS

....

....

....

HOW DO I FEEL?(A.M.) ☺ ☹ 😐   HOW DO I FEEL?(P.M.) ☺ ☹ 😐

ENERGY LEVEL ❶ ❷ ❸ ❹ ❺   ENERGY LEVEL ❶ ❷ ❸ ❹ ❺

🌅 SUN & FRESH AIR ....   🖥 SCREEN TIME ....

ON A CLEANSE? Y / N   ALCOHOL 🍷 🍷 🍷 🍷 🍷 🍷

TODAY'S DIET:

✕ FOOD LOG ✕

BREAKFAST	LUNCH	DINNER	SNACK

WATER INTAKE 🌢🌢🌢🌢🌢🌢🌢🌢 TOTAL CALORIES:

◀▬▶ EXERCISE LOG ◀▬▶

(OPTIONAL) WEIGHT:				START TIME	END TIME
STRETCH 🧘					

WEIGHT TRAINING 🏋	WEIGHT	SETS	REPS	START TIME	END TIME

CARDIO 🏃	START TIME	END TIME

Circle how you feel today or write your own:...

Kind	Connected	Clear	Playful	Simple	Abundant
Purposeful	Calm	Loving	Joyful		Adventurous
Open	Spiritual	Free	Faithful		Generous

What did you learn today?

I AM CONFIDENT.

DATE: M   T   W   TH   F   S   S

WEEK # 9   TOTAL HOURS SLEPT:

TONIGHT'S BEDTIME GOAL:

♥ TODAY, I AM GRATEFUL FOR:

🧘 SELF-CARE GOAL(S):

PRAYER REQUEST:

⚔ PERSONAL AFFIRMATION:

⚡ VITAMINS, SUPPLEMENTS & MEDICATIONS

....

....

....   🖊 HEALTH SYMPTOMS

....

....

....

HOW DO I FEEL?(A.M.) ☺ ☹ 😐   HOW DO I FEEL?(P.M.) ☺ ☹ 😐

ENERGY LEVEL ❶ ❷ ❸ ❹ ❺   ENERGY LEVEL ❶ ❷ ❸ ❹ ❺

☀ SUN & FRESH AIR ....   🖥 SCREEN TIME ....

ON A CLEANSE? Y / N   ALCOHOL 🍷 🍷 🍷 🍷 🍷

TODAY'S DIET:

✖ FOOD LOG ✖			
BREAKFAST	LUNCH	DINNER	SNACK

WATER INTAKE 🔸🔸🔸🔸🔸🔸🔸🔸 TOTAL CALORIES:

◁—◻ EXERCISE LOG ◻—▷

(OPTIONAL) WEIGHT:				START TIME	END TIME
STRETCH 🧘					

WEIGHT TRAINING 🏋	WEIGHT	SETS	REPS	START TIME	END TIME

CARDIO 🏃	START TIME	END TIME

Circle how you feel today or write your own: ....

Kind	Connected	Clear	Playful	Simple	Abundant
Purposeful	Calm	Loving	Joyful		Adventurous
Open	Spiritual	Free	Faithful		Generous

What did you learn today?

NOTES

_____

_____

_____

_____

_____

_____

_____

_____

_____

_____

_____

_____

_____

WELLNESS APPOINTMENTS:

_____

_____

NEEDS IMPROVEMENT:

_____

_____

INSIGHTS & LESSONS:

_____

_____

SUCCESSES & WINS:

_____

_____

_____

I AM FEARLESS.

DATE: M   T   W   TH   F   S   S

WEEK # 10   TOTAL HOURS SLEPT:

TONIGHT'S BEDTIME GOAL:

♥ TODAY, I AM GRATEFUL FOR:

🧘 SELF-CARE GOAL(S):

PRAYER REQUEST:

⚔ PERSONAL AFFIRMATION:

🔋 VITAMINS, SUPPLEMENTS & MEDICATIONS

....

....

....   🌡 HEALTH SYMPTOMS

....

....

....

HOW DO I FEEL?(A.M.) ☺ ☹ 😐   HOW DO I FEEL?(P.M.) ☺ ☹ 😐

ENERGY LEVEL ❶ ❷ ❸ ❹ ❺   ENERGY LEVEL ❶ ❷ ❸ ❹ ❺

🌅 SUN & FRESH AIR ....   🖥 SCREEN TIME ....

ON A CLEANSE? Y / N   ALCOHOL 🍷 🍷 🍷 🍷 🍷

TODAY'S DIET:

✖ FOOD LOG ✖

BREAKFAST	LUNCH	DINNER	SNACK

WATER INTAKE 🌢🌢🌢🌢🌢🌢🌢🌢 TOTAL CALORIES:

EXERCISE LOG					

(OPTIONAL) WEIGHT:				START TIME	END TIME
STRETCH					
WEIGHT TRAINING	WEIGHT	SETS	REPS	START TIME	END TIME

CARDIO		START TIME	END TIME

Circle how you feel today or write your own: ....

Kind   Connected   Clear   Playful   Simple   Abundant

Purposeful   Calm   Loving   Joyful   Adventurous

Open   Spiritual   Free   Faithful   Generous

What did you learn today?

I AM WORTHY.

DATE: M   T   W   TH   F   S   S

WEEK # 10   TOTAL HOURS SLEPT:

TONIGHT'S BEDTIME GOAL:

♥ TODAY, I AM GRATEFUL FOR:

🧘 SELF-CARE GOAL(S):

PRAYER REQUEST:

⚔ PERSONAL AFFIRMATION:

⚡ VITAMINS, SUPPLEMENTS & MEDICATIONS

....

....

....   🖊 HEALTH SYMPTOMS

....

....

....

HOW DO I FEEL?(A.M.) ☺ ☹ 😐   HOW DO I FEEL?(P.M.) ☺ ☹ 😐

ENERGY LEVEL ①–②–③–④–⑤   ENERGY LEVEL ①–②–③–④–⑤

☀ SUN & FRESH AIR ....   🖥 SCREEN TIME ....

ON A CLEANSE? Y / N   ALCOHOL 🍷 🍷 🍷 🍷 🍷 🍷

TODAY'S DIET:

✗ FOOD LOG ✗

BREAKFAST	LUNCH	DINNER	SNACK

WATER INTAKE 🩸🩸🩸🩸🩸🩸🩸🩸 TOTAL CALORIES:

⟨⊨⊟ EXERCISE LOG ⊨⊟⟩

(OPTIONAL) WEIGHT:				START TIME	END TIME
STRETCH					
WEIGHT TRAINING	WEIGHT	SETS	REPS	START TIME	END TIME

CARDIO		START TIME	END TIME

Circle how you feel today or write your own: ....

Kind	Connected	Clear	Playful	Simple	Abundant
Purposeful	Calm	Loving	Joyful		Adventurous
Open	Spiritual	Free	Faithful		Generous

What did you learn today?

I AM POWERFUL.

DATE: M   T   W   TH   F   S   S

WEEK # 10   TOTAL HOURS SLEPT:

TONIGHT'S BEDTIME GOAL:

♥ TODAY, I AM GRATEFUL FOR:

🧘 SELF-CARE GOAL(S):

PRAYER REQUEST:

⚔ PERSONAL AFFIRMATION:

🔋 VITAMINS, SUPPLEMENTS & MEDICATIONS

....

....

....   🖊 HEALTH SYMPTOMS

....

....

....

HOW DO I FEEL?(A.M.) 😊 ☹ 😐   HOW DO I FEEL?(P.M.) 😊 ☹ 😐

ENERGY LEVEL ① ② ③ ④ ⑤   ENERGY LEVEL ① ② ③ ④ ⑤

☀ SUN & FRESH AIR ....   🖥 SCREEN TIME ....

ON A CLEANSE? Y / N   ALCOHOL 🍷 🍷 🍷 🍷 🍷

TODAY'S DIET:

✗ FOOD LOG ✗

BREAKFAST	LUNCH	DINNER	SNACK

WATER INTAKE 🔴🔴🔴🔴🔴🔴🔴🔴   TOTAL CALORIES:

◧—◍ EXERCISE LOG ◧—◍

(OPTIONAL) WEIGHT:				START TIME	END TIME
STRETCH 🧘					

WEIGHT TRAINING 🏋️	WEIGHT	SETS	REPS	START TIME	END TIME

CARDIO 🏃	START TIME	END TIME

Circle how you feel today or write your own: ....

Kind	Connected	Clear	Playful	Simple	Abundant
Purposeful	Calm	Loving	Joyful		Adventurous
Open	Spiritual	Free	Faithful		Generous

What did you learn today?

I AM THANKFUL

DATE: M   T   W   TH   F   S   S

WEEK # 10   TOTAL HOURS SLEPT:

TONIGHT'S BEDTIME GOAL:

❤ TODAY, I AM GRATEFUL FOR:

🧘 SELF-CARE GOAL(S):

PRAYER REQUEST:

⚔ PERSONAL AFFIRMATION:

🔋 VITAMINS, SUPPLEMENTS & MEDICATIONS

....

....

....

....

....

....

✎ HEALTH SYMPTOMS

HOW DO I FEEL?(A.M.) ☺ ☹ 😐   HOW DO I FEEL?(P.M.) ☺ ☹ 😐

ENERGY LEVEL ❶ ❷ ❸ ❹ ❺   ENERGY LEVEL ❶ ❷ ❸ ❹ ❺

🌅 SUN & FRESH AIR ....   📱 SCREEN TIME ....

ON A CLEANSE? Y / N   ALCOHOL 🍷 🍷 🍷 🍷 🍷

TODAY'S DIET:

✖ FOOD LOG ✖

BREAKFAST	LUNCH	DINNER	SNACK

WATER INTAKE 🔴🔴🔴🔴🔴🔴🔴🔴 TOTAL CALORIES:

⬤—▮ EXERCISE LOG ▮—⬤					

(OPTIONAL) WEIGHT:				START TIME	END TIME
STRETCH					

WEIGHT TRAINING	WEIGHT	SETS	REPS	START TIME	END TIME

CARDIO			START TIME	END TIME

Circle how you feel today or write your own: ....

| Kind | Connected | Clear | Playful | Simple | Abundant |

| Purposeful | Calm | Loving | Joyful | Adventurous |

| Open | Spiritual | Free | Faithful | Generous |

What did you learn today?

I AM BLESSED.

DATE: M   T   W   TH   F   S   S

WEEK # 10   TOTAL HOURS SLEPT:

TONIGHT'S BEDTIME GOAL:

♥ TODAY, I AM GRATEFUL FOR:

🧘 SELF-CARE GOAL(S):

PRAYER REQUEST:

⚔ PERSONAL AFFIRMATION:

⚡ VITAMINS, SUPPLEMENTS & MEDICATIONS

....

....

.... 🖊 HEALTH SYMPTOMS

....

....

....

HOW DO I FEEL?(A.M.) ☺ ☹ 😐   HOW DO I FEEL?(P.M.) ☺ ☹ 😐

ENERGY LEVEL ❶ ❷ ❸ ❹ ❺   ENERGY LEVEL ❶ ❷ ❸ ❹ ❺

☀ SUN & FRESH AIR ....   💻 SCREEN TIME ....

ON A CLEANSE?   Y / N   ALCOHOL 🍷 🍷 🍷 🍷 🍷

TODAY'S DIET:

✖ FOOD LOG ✖

BREAKFAST	LUNCH	DINNER	SNACK

WATER INTAKE 🔻🔻🔻🔻🔻🔻🔻🔻 TOTAL CALORIES:

◁—◻ EXERCISE LOG ◻—▷

(OPTIONAL) WEIGHT:				START TIME	END TIME
STRETCH					

WEIGHT TRAINING	WEIGHT	SETS	REPS	START TIME	END TIME

CARDIO		START TIME	END TIME

Circle how you feel today or write your own: ....

Kind	Connected	Clear	Playful	Simple	Abundant
Purposeful	Calm	Loving	Joyful		Adventurous
Open	Spiritual	Free	Faithful		Generous

What did you learn today?

I AM BRAVE.

DATE:		M	T	W	TH	F	S	S

WEEK # 10   TOTAL HOURS SLEPT:

TONIGHT'S BEDTIME GOAL:

♥ TODAY, I AM GRATEFUL FOR:

🧘 SELF-CARE GOAL(S):

PRAYER REQUEST:

✕ PERSONAL AFFIRMATION:

⚡ VITAMINS, SUPPLEMENTS & MEDICATIONS

....
....
....   🖊 HEALTH SYMPTOMS
....
....

HOW DO I FEEL?(A.M.) ☺ ☹ 😐   HOW DO I FEEL?(P.M.) ☺ ☹ 😐

ENERGY LEVEL ❶ ❷ ❸ ❹ ❺   ENERGY LEVEL ❶ ❷ ❸ ❹ ❺

☀ SUN & FRESH AIR ....   🖥 SCREEN TIME ....

ON A CLEANSE? Y / N   ALCOHOL 🍷 🍷 🍷 🍷 🍷

TODAY'S DIET:

✕ FOOD LOG ✕

BREAKFAST	LUNCH	DINNER	SNACK

WATER INTAKE 🔴🔴🔴🔴🔴🔴🔴🔴 TOTAL CALORIES:

⬤—⬤ EXERCISE LOG ⬤—⬤

(OPTIONAL) WEIGHT:				START TIME	END TIME
STRETCH					
WEIGHT TRAINING	WEIGHT	SETS	REPS	START TIME	END TIME

CARDIO	START TIME	END TIME

Circle how you feel today or write your own: ....

Kind　　　Connected　　　Clear　　　Playful　　　Simple　　　Abundant

Purposeful　　　Calm　　　Loving　　　Joyful　　　Adventurous

Open　　　Spiritual　　　Free　　　Faithful　　　Generous

What did you learn today?

I AM CONFIDENT.

DATE: M   T   W   TH   F   S   S

WEEK # 10   TOTAL HOURS SLEPT:

TONIGHT'S BEDTIME GOAL:

♥ TODAY, I AM GRATEFUL FOR:

🧘 SELF-CARE GOAL(S):

PRAYER REQUEST:

⚔ PERSONAL AFFIRMATION:

⚡ VITAMINS, SUPPLEMENTS & MEDICATIONS

....

....

....   🖊 HEALTH SYMPTOMS

....

....

....

HOW DO I FEEL?(A.M.) ☺ ☹ 😐   HOW DO I FEEL?(P.M.) ☺ ☹ 😐

ENERGY LEVEL ➊ ➋ ➌ ➍ ➎   ENERGY LEVEL ➊ ➋ ➌ ➍ ➎

🌅 SUN & FRESH AIR ....   🖥 SCREEN TIME ....

ON A CLEANSE? Y / N   ALCOHOL 🍷 🍷 🍷 🍷 🍷

TODAY'S DIET:

✗ FOOD LOG ✗

BREAKFAST	LUNCH	DINNER	SNACK

WATER INTAKE 🔴🔴🔴🔴🔴🔴🔴🔴 TOTAL CALORIES:

⬦—⬧ EXERCISE LOG ⬦—⬧

(OPTIONAL) WEIGHT:				START TIME	END TIME
STRETCH					
WEIGHT TRAINING	WEIGHT	SETS	REPS	START TIME	END TIME

CARDIO		START TIME	END TIME

Circle how you feel today or write your own:...

Kind	Connected	Clear	Playful	Simple	Abundant
Purposeful	Calm	Loving	Joyful		Adventurous
Open	Spiritual	Free	Faithful		Generous

What did you learn today?

NOTES

_____

_____

_____

_____

_____

_____

_____

_____

_____

_____

_____

_____

_____

WELLNESS APPOINTMENTS:

_____

_____

NEEDS IMPROVEMENT:

_____

_____

INSIGHTS & LESSONS:

_____

_____

SUCCESSES & WINS:

_____

_____

_____

I AM FEARLESS.

DATE:		M	T	W	TH	F	S	S

WEEK # 11   TOTAL HOURS SLEPT:

TONIGHT'S BEDTIME GOAL:

♥ TODAY, I AM GRATEFUL FOR:

🧘 SELF-CARE GOAL(S):

PRAYER REQUEST:

⚔ PERSONAL AFFIRMATION:

🔋 VITAMINS, SUPPLEMENTS & MEDICATIONS

....

....

....   🖊 HEALTH SYMPTOMS

....

....

....

HOW DO I FEEL?(A.M.) ☺ ☹ 😐   HOW DO I FEEL?(P.M.) ☺ ☹ 😐

ENERGY LEVEL ❶ ❷ ❸ ❹ ❺   ENERGY LEVEL ❶ ❷ ❸ ❹ ❺

☀ SUN & FRESH AIR ....   🖥 SCREEN TIME ....

ON A CLEANSE? Y / N   ALCOHOL 🍷 🍷 🍷 🍷 🍷

TODAY'S DIET:

✖ FOOD LOG ✖

BREAKFAST	LUNCH	DINNER	SNACK

WATER INTAKE 🌢🌢🌢🌢🌢🌢🌢🌢 TOTAL CALORIES:

⬤━⬤ EXERCISE LOG ⬤━⬤					

(OPTIONAL) WEIGHT:				START TIME	END TIME
STRETCH 🧘					
WEIGHT TRAINING 🏋	WEIGHT	SETS	REPS	START TIME	END TIME
CARDIO 🚶				START TIME	END TIME

Circle how you feel today or write your own: ....

Kind   Connected   Clear   Playful   Simple   Abundant

Purposeful   Calm   Loving   Joyful   Adventurous

Open   Spiritual   Free   Faithful   Generous

What did you learn today?

I AM WORTHY

DATE: M   T   W   TH   F   S   S

WEEK # 11   TOTAL HOURS SLEPT:

TONIGHT'S BEDTIME GOAL:

♥ TODAY, I AM GRATEFUL FOR:

🧘 SELF-CARE GOAL(S):

PRAYER REQUEST:

⚔ PERSONAL AFFIRMATION:

⚡ VITAMINS, SUPPLEMENTS & MEDICATIONS

....

....

.... ### 🖊 HEALTH SYMPTOMS

....

....

....

HOW DO I FEEL?(A.M.) ☺ ☹ 😐   HOW DO I FEEL?(P.M.) ☺ ☹ 😐

ENERGY LEVEL ❶ ❷ ❸ ❹ ❺   ENERGY LEVEL ❶ ❷ ❸ ❹ ❺

🌅 SUN & FRESH AIR ....   📱 SCREEN TIME ....

ON A CLEANSE? Y / N   ALCOHOL 🍷 🍷 🍷 🍷 🍷

TODAY'S DIET:

✖ FOOD LOG ✖

BREAKFAST	LUNCH	DINNER	SNACK

WATER INTAKE ♦♦♦♦♦♦♦♦ TOTAL CALORIES:

◧─◻ EXERCISE LOG ◧─◻

(OPTIONAL) WEIGHT:				START TIME	END TIME
STRETCH 🧘					

WEIGHT TRAINING 🏋	WEIGHT	SETS	REPS	START TIME	END TIME

CARDIO 🏃				START TIME	END TIME

Circle how you feel today or write your own: ....

Kind	Connected	Clear	Playful	Simple	Abundant
Purposeful	Calm	Loving	Joyful		Adventurous
Open	Spiritual	Free	Faithful		Generous

What did you learn today?

I AM POWERFUL.

DATE: M   T   W   TH   F   S   S

WEEK # 11   TOTAL HOURS SLEPT:

TONIGHT'S BEDTIME GOAL:

♥ TODAY, I AM GRATEFUL FOR:

🧘 SELF-CARE GOAL(S):

PRAYER REQUEST:

⚔ PERSONAL AFFIRMATION:

🔋 VITAMINS, SUPPLEMENTS & MEDICATIONS

....
....
....   🌡 HEALTH SYMPTOMS
....
....
....

HOW DO I FEEL?(A.M.) ☺ ☹ 😐   HOW DO I FEEL?(P.M.) ☺ ☹ 😐

ENERGY LEVEL ❶ ❷ ❸ ❹ ❺   ENERGY LEVEL ❶ ❷ ❸ ❹ ❺

🌅 SUN & FRESH AIR ....   📱 SCREEN TIME ....

ON A CLEANSE? Y / N   ALCOHOL 🍷 🍷 🍷 🍷 🍷

TODAY'S DIET:

✖ FOOD LOG ✖

BREAKFAST	LUNCH	DINNER	SNACK

WATER INTAKE 💧💧💧💧💧💧💧💧 TOTAL CALORIES:

◁—▷ EXERCISE LOG ◁—▷

(OPTIONAL) WEIGHT:				START TIME	END TIME
STRETCH					

WEIGHT TRAINING	WEIGHT	SETS	REPS	START TIME	END TIME

CARDIO	START TIME	END TIME

Circle how you feel today or write your own:...

Kind	Connected	Clear	Playful	Simple	Abundant
Purposeful	Calm	Loving	Joyful		Adventurous
Open	Spiritual	Free	Faithful		Generous

What did you learn today?

I AM THANKFUL

DATE: M   T   W   TH   F   S   S

WEEK # 11   TOTAL HOURS SLEPT:

TONIGHT'S BEDTIME GOAL:

♥ TODAY, I AM GRATEFUL FOR:

🧘 SELF-CARE GOAL(S):

PRAYER REQUEST:

⚔ PERSONAL AFFIRMATION:

🔋 VITAMINS, SUPPLEMENTS & MEDICATIONS

....
....
....   🌡 HEALTH SYMPTOMS
....
....
....

HOW DO I FEEL?(A.M.) ☺ ☹ 😐   HOW DO I FEEL?(P.M.) ☺ ☹ 😐

ENERGY LEVEL ❶ ❷ ❸ ❹ ❺   ENERGY LEVEL ❶ ❷ ❸ ❹ ❺

🌅 SUN & FRESH AIR ....   🖥 SCREEN TIME ....

ON A CLEANSE? Y / N   ALCOHOL 🍷 🍷 🍷 🍷 🍷

TODAY'S DIET:

✖ FOOD LOG ✖

BREAKFAST	LUNCH	DINNER	SNACK

WATER INTAKE 🔻🔻🔻🔻🔻🔻🔻🔻 TOTAL CALORIES:

◖—◗ EXERCISE LOG ◖—◗

(OPTIONAL) WEIGHT:				START TIME	END TIME
STRETCH					

WEIGHT TRAINING	WEIGHT	SETS	REPS	START TIME	END TIME

CARDIO	START TIME	END TIME

Circle how you feel today or write your own: ....

Kind	Connected	Clear	Playful	Simple	Abundant
Purposeful	Calm	Loving	Joyful		Adventurous
Open	Spiritual	Free	Faithful		Generous

What did you learn today?

I AM BLESSED.

DATE: M   T   W   TH   F   S   S

WEEK # 11   TOTAL HOURS SLEPT:

TONIGHT'S BEDTIME GOAL:

♥ TODAY, I AM GRATEFUL FOR:

🧘 SELF-CARE GOAL(S):

PRAYER REQUEST:

⚔ PERSONAL AFFIRMATION:

⚡ VITAMINS, SUPPLEMENTS & MEDICATIONS

....

....

....   ✏ HEALTH SYMPTOMS

....

....

....

HOW DO I FEEL?(A.M.) ☺ ☹ 😐   HOW DO I FEEL?(P.M.) ☺ ☹ 😐

ENERGY LEVEL ❶ ❷ ❸ ❹ ❺   ENERGY LEVEL ❶ ❷ ❸ ❹ ❺

🌅 SUN & FRESH AIR ....   🖥 SCREEN TIME ....

ON A CLEANSE?   Y / N   ALCOHOL 🍷 🍷 🍷 🍷 🍷

TODAY'S DIET:

✗ FOOD LOG ✗

BREAKFAST	LUNCH	DINNER	SNACK

WATER INTAKE 🔴🔴🔴🔴🔴🔴🔴🔴 TOTAL CALORIES:

◁━▷ EXERCISE LOG ◁━▷					

(OPTIONAL) WEIGHT:				START TIME	END TIME
STRETCH					

WEIGHT TRAINING	WEIGHT	SETS	REPS	START TIME	END TIME

CARDIO		START TIME	END TIME

Circle how you feel today or write your own: ....

Kind   Connected   Clear   Playful   Simple   Abundant

Purposeful   Calm   Loving   Joyful   Adventurous

Open   Spiritual   Free   Faithful   Generous

What did you learn today?

I AM BRAVE.

DATE:		M	T	W	TH	F	S	S

WEEK # 11   TOTAL HOURS SLEPT:

TONIGHT'S BEDTIME GOAL:

♥ TODAY, I AM GRATEFUL FOR:

🧘 SELF-CARE GOAL(S):

PRAYER REQUEST:

⚔ PERSONAL AFFIRMATION:

🔋 VITAMINS, SUPPLEMENTS & MEDICATIONS

....
....
.... ✎ HEALTH SYMPTOMS
....
....
....

HOW DO I FEEL?(A.M.) ☺ ☹ 😐   HOW DO I FEEL?(P.M.) ☺ ☹ 😐

ENERGY LEVEL ❶ ❷ ❸ ❹ ❺   ENERGY LEVEL ❶ ❷ ❸ ❹ ❺

☀ SUN & FRESH AIR ....   🖥 SCREEN TIME ....

ON A CLEANSE? Y / N   ALCOHOL 🍷 🍷 🍷 🍷 🍷

TODAY'S DIET:

✖ FOOD LOG ✖

BREAKFAST	LUNCH	DINNER	SNACK

WATER INTAKE 🌢🌢🌢🌢🌢🌢🌢🌢 TOTAL CALORIES:

◁▭▷ EXERCISE LOG ◁▭▷

(OPTIONAL) WEIGHT:				START TIME	END TIME
STRETCH					

WEIGHT TRAINING	WEIGHT	SETS	REPS	START TIME	END TIME

CARDIO	START TIME	END TIME

Circle how you feel today or write your own: ....

Kind	Connected	Clear	Playful	Simple	Abundant
Purposeful	Calm	Loving	Joyful		Adventurous
Open	Spiritual	Free	Faithful		Generous

What did you learn today?

I AM CONFIDENT.

DATE: M   T   W   TH   F   S   S

WEEK # 11   TOTAL HOURS SLEPT:

TONIGHT'S BEDTIME GOAL:

♥ TODAY, I AM GRATEFUL FOR:

🧘 SELF-CARE GOAL(S):

PRAYER REQUEST:

⚔ PERSONAL AFFIRMATION:

⚡ VITAMINS, SUPPLEMENTS & MEDICATIONS

....

....   🖊 HEALTH SYMPTOMS

....

....

....

HOW DO I FEEL?(A.M.) 😊 😞 😐   HOW DO I FEEL?(P.M.) 😊 😞 😐

ENERGY LEVEL ❶ ❷ ❸ ❹ ❺   ENERGY LEVEL ❶ ❷ ❸ ❹ ❺

☀ SUN & FRESH AIR ....   🖥 SCREEN TIME ....

ON A CLEANSE? Y / N   ALCOHOL 🍷 🍷 🍷 🍷 🍷

TODAY'S DIET:

✗ FOOD LOG ✗

BREAKFAST	LUNCH	DINNER	SNACK

WATER INTAKE 🔻🔻🔻🔻🔻🔻🔻🔻 TOTAL CALORIES:

◁▭▷ EXERCISE LOG ◁▭▷

(OPTIONAL) WEIGHT:				START TIME	END TIME
STRETCH					

WEIGHT TRAINING	WEIGHT	SETS	REPS	START TIME	END TIME

CARDIO	START TIME	END TIME

Circle how you feel today or write your own: ....

Kind	Connected	Clear	Playful	Simple	Abundant
Purposeful	Calm	Loving	Joyful		Adventurous
Open	Spiritual	Free	Faithful		Generous

What did you learn today?

_____

_____

_____

_____

_____

_____

_____

_____

_____

_____

_____

_____

_____

WELLNESS APPOINTMENTS:

_____

_____

NEEDS IMPROVEMENT:

_____

_____

INSIGHTS & LESSONS:

_____

_____

SUCCESSES & WINS:

_____

_____

I AM FEARLESS.

DATE: M   T   W   TH   F   S   S

WEEK # 12   TOTAL HOURS SLEPT:

TONIGHT'S BEDTIME GOAL:

♥ TODAY, I AM GRATEFUL FOR:

🧘 SELF-CARE GOAL(S):

PRAYER REQUEST:

⚔ PERSONAL AFFIRMATION:

🔋 VITAMINS, SUPPLEMENTS & MEDICATIONS

....

....   🖊 HEALTH SYMPTOMS

....

....

....

....

HOW DO I FEEL?(A.M.) ☺ ☹ 😐   HOW DO I FEEL?(P.M.) ☺ ☹ 😐

ENERGY LEVEL ❶ ❷ ❸ ❹ ❺   ENERGY LEVEL ❶ ❷ ❸ ❹ ❺

🌅 SUN & FRESH AIR ....   🖥 SCREEN TIME ....

ON A CLEANSE? Y / N   ALCOHOL 🍷 🍷 🍷 🍷 🍷

TODAY'S DIET:

✕ FOOD LOG ✕

BREAKFAST	LUNCH	DINNER	SNACK

WATER INTAKE 🔴🔴🔴🔴🔴🔴🔴🔴 TOTAL CALORIES:

⫸—⫸ EXERCISE LOG ⫸—⫸

(OPTIONAL) WEIGHT:				START TIME	END TIME
STRETCH 🧘					

WEIGHT TRAINING 🏋	WEIGHT	SETS	REPS	START TIME	END TIME

CARDIO 🏃		START TIME	END TIME

Circle how you feel today or write your own: ....

Kind	Connected	Clear	Playful	Simple	Abundant
Purposeful	Calm	Loving	Joyful		Adventurous
Open	Spiritual	Free	Faithful		Generous

What did you learn today?

☀ ☽ ☐

I AM WORTHY.

☀ ☽

DATE: M   T   W   TH   F   S   S

WEEK # 12   TOTAL HOURS SLEPT:

TONIGHT'S BEDTIME GOAL:

♥ TODAY, I AM GRATEFUL FOR:

🧘 SELF-CARE GOAL(S):

PRAYER REQUEST:

⚔ PERSONAL AFFIRMATION:

⚡ VITAMINS, SUPPLEMENTS & MEDICATIONS

....

....

                         🖊 HEALTH SYMPTOMS

....

....

....

HOW DO I FEEL?(A.M.) ☺ ☹ 😐   HOW DO I FEEL?(P.M.) ☺ ☹ 😐

ENERGY LEVEL ❶ ❷ ❸ ❹ ❺   ENERGY LEVEL ❶ ❷ ❸ ❹ ❺

☀ SUN & FRESH AIR ....   🖥 SCREEN TIME ....

ON A CLEANSE? Y / N   ALCOHOL 🍷 🍷 🍷 🍷 🍷

TODAY'S DIET:

✗ FOOD LOG ✗

BREAKFAST	LUNCH	DINNER	SNACK

WATER INTAKE 🌑🌑🌑🌑🌑🌑🌑🌑 TOTAL CALORIES:

⬛—◻ EXERCISE LOG ◻—⬛

(OPTIONAL) WEIGHT:				START TIME	END TIME
STRETCH 🧘					

WEIGHT TRAINING 🏋	WEIGHT	SETS	REPS	START TIME	END TIME

CARDIO 🏃		START TIME	END TIME

Circle how you feel today or write your own: ....

Kind	Connected	Clear	Playful	Simple	Abundant
Purposeful	Calm	Loving	Joyful		Adventurous
Open	Spiritual	Free	Faithful		Generous

What did you learn today?

I AM POWERFUL.

DATE: M   T   W   TH   F   S   S

WEEK # 12   TOTAL HOURS SLEPT:

TONIGHT'S BEDTIME GOAL:

❤ TODAY, I AM GRATEFUL FOR:

🧘 SELF-CARE GOAL(S):

PRAYER REQUEST:

⚔ PERSONAL AFFIRMATION:

⚡ VITAMINS, SUPPLEMENTS & MEDICATIONS

....

....

.... 🖊 HEALTH SYMPTOMS

....

....

....

HOW DO I FEEL?(A.M.) ☺ ☹ 😐   HOW DO I FEEL?(P.M.) ☺ ☹ 😐

ENERGY LEVEL ❶ ❷ ❸ ❹ ❺   ENERGY LEVEL ❶ ❷ ❸ ❹ ❺

🌅 SUN & FRESH AIR ....   💻 SCREEN TIME ....

ON A CLEANSE?   Y / N   ALCOHOL 🍷 🍷 🍷 🍷 🍷

TODAY'S DIET:

✖ FOOD LOG ✖

BREAKFAST	LUNCH	DINNER	SNACK

WATER INTAKE 💧💧💧💧💧💧💧💧   TOTAL CALORIES:

◖—◗ EXERCISE LOG ◖—◗

(OPTIONAL) WEIGHT:				START TIME	END TIME
STRETCH					

WEIGHT TRAINING	WEIGHT	SETS	REPS	START TIME	END TIME

CARDIO		START TIME	END TIME

Circle how you feel today or write your own: ....

Kind	Connected	Clear	Playful	Simple	Abundant
Purposeful	Calm	Loving	Joyful		Adventurous
Open	Spiritual	Free	Faithful		Generous

What did you learn today?

I AM THANKFUL.

DATE: M   T   W   TH   F   S   S

WEEK # 12   TOTAL HOURS SLEPT:

TONIGHT'S BEDTIME GOAL:

♥ TODAY, I AM GRATEFUL FOR:

🧘 SELF-CARE GOAL(S):

PRAYER REQUEST:

⚔ PERSONAL AFFIRMATION:

🔋 VITAMINS, SUPPLEMENTS & MEDICATIONS

....

....

....   🖊 HEALTH SYMPTOMS

....

....

....

HOW DO I FEEL?(A.M.) 🙂 ☹ 😐   HOW DO I FEEL?(P.M.) 🙂 ☹ 😐

ENERGY LEVEL ❶ ❷ ❸ ❹ ❺   ENERGY LEVEL ❶ ❷ ❸ ❹ ❺

☀ SUN & FRESH AIR ....   💻 SCREEN TIME ....

ON A CLEANSE? Y / N   ALCOHOL 🍷 🍷 🍷 🍷 🍷

TODAY'S DIET:

✕ FOOD LOG ✕

BREAKFAST	LUNCH	DINNER	SNACK

WATER INTAKE 🔹🔹🔹🔹🔹🔹🔹🔹 TOTAL CALORIES:

◁━▷ EXERCISE LOG ◁━▷

(OPTIONAL) WEIGHT:				START TIME	END TIME
STRETCH					

WEIGHT TRAINING	WEIGHT	SETS	REPS	START TIME	END TIME

CARDIO	START TIME	END TIME

Circle how you feel today or write your own: ....

Kind   Connected   Clear   Playful   Simple   Abundant

Purposeful   Calm   Loving   Joyful   Adventurous

Open   Spiritual   Free   Faithful   Generous

What did you learn today?

I AM BLESSED.

DATE:		M	T	W	TH	F	S	S

WEEK # 12   TOTAL HOURS SLEPT:

TONIGHT'S BEDTIME GOAL:

♥ TODAY, I AM GRATEFUL FOR:

🧘 SELF-CARE GOAL(S):

PRAYER REQUEST:

⚔ PERSONAL AFFIRMATION:

⚡ VITAMINS, SUPPLEMENTS & MEDICATIONS

....
....
....   ✏ HEALTH SYMPTOMS
....
....
....

HOW DO I FEEL?(A.M.) ☺ ☹ 😐   HOW DO I FEEL?(P.M.) ☺ ☹ 😐

ENERGY LEVEL ❶ ❷ ❸ ❹ ❺   ENERGY LEVEL ❶ ❷ ❸ ❹ ❺

☀ SUN & FRESH AIR ....   💻 SCREEN TIME ....

ON A CLEANSE? Y / N   ALCOHOL 🍷 🍷 🍷 🍷 🍷

TODAY'S DIET:

✕ FOOD LOG ✕

BREAKFAST	LUNCH	DINNER	SNACK

WATER INTAKE 🔹🔹🔹🔹🔹🔹🔹🔹 TOTAL CALORIES:

⫟—⫟ EXERCISE LOG ⫟—⫟					

(OPTIONAL) WEIGHT:				START TIME	END TIME
STRETCH					

WEIGHT TRAINING	WEIGHT	SETS	REPS	START TIME	END TIME

CARDIO		START TIME	END TIME

Circle how you feel today or write your own: ....

Kind	Connected	Clear	Playful	Simple	Abundant
Purposeful	Calm	Loving	Joyful		Adventurous
Open	Spiritual	Free	Faithful		Generous

What did you learn today?

I AM BRAVE.

DATE: M   T   W   TH   F   S   S

WEEK # 12   TOTAL HOURS SLEPT:

TONIGHT'S BEDTIME GOAL:

♥ TODAY, I AM GRATEFUL FOR:

🧘 SELF-CARE GOAL(S):

PRAYER REQUEST:

⚔ PERSONAL AFFIRMATION:

🔋 VITAMINS, SUPPLEMENTS & MEDICATIONS

....

....

....   🖊 HEALTH SYMPTOMS

....

....

....

HOW DO I FEEL?(A.M.) ☺ ☹ 😐   HOW DO I FEEL?(P.M.) ☺ ☹ 😐

ENERGY LEVEL ❶ ❷ ❸ ❹ ❺   ENERGY LEVEL ❶ ❷ ❸ ❹ ❺

🌅 SUN & FRESH AIR ....   📱 SCREEN TIME ....

ON A CLEANSE?   Y / N   ALCOHOL 🍷 🍷 🍷 🍷 🍷

TODAY'S DIET:

✗ FOOD LOG ✗

BREAKFAST	LUNCH	DINNER	SNACK

WATER INTAKE 🌢🌢🌢🌢🌢🌢🌢🌢 TOTAL CALORIES:

◫—◫ EXERCISE LOG ◫—◫

(OPTIONAL) WEIGHT:				START TIME	END TIME
STRETCH					
WEIGHT TRAINING	WEIGHT	SETS	REPS	START TIME	END TIME
CARDIO				START TIME	END TIME

Circle how you feel today or write your own: ....

| Kind | Connected | Clear | Playful | Simple | Abundant |

| Purposeful | Calm | Loving | Joyful | Adventurous |

| Open | Spiritual | Free | Faithful | Generous |

What did you learn today?

I AM CONFIDENT.

DATE:	M	T	W	TH	F	S	S

WEEK # 12   TOTAL HOURS SLEPT:

TONIGHT'S BEDTIME GOAL:

♥ TODAY, I AM GRATEFUL FOR:

🧘 SELF-CARE GOAL(S):

PRAYER REQUEST:

⚔ PERSONAL AFFIRMATION:

🔋 VITAMINS, SUPPLEMENTS & MEDICATIONS

....

....

....   🌡 HEALTH SYMPTOMS

....

....

....

HOW DO I FEEL?(A.M.) ☺ ☹ 😐   HOW DO I FEEL?(P.M.) ☺ ☹ 😐

ENERGY LEVEL ① ② ③ ④ ⑤   ENERGY LEVEL ① ② ③ ④ ⑤

🌅 SUN & FRESH AIR ....   💻 SCREEN TIME ....

ON A CLEANSE? Y / N   ALCOHOL 🍷 🍷 🍷 🍷 🍷 🍷

TODAY'S DIET:

✖ FOOD LOG ✖

BREAKFAST	LUNCH	DINNER	SNACK

WATER INTAKE 💧💧💧💧💧💧💧💧 TOTAL CALORIES:

⊪—⊪ EXERCISE LOG ⊪—⊪

(OPTIONAL) WEIGHT:				START TIME	END TIME
STRETCH					

WEIGHT TRAINING	WEIGHT	SETS	REPS	START TIME	END TIME

CARDIO	START TIME	END TIME

Circle how you feel today or write your own: ....

Kind	Connected	Clear	Playful	Simple	Abundant

Purposeful	Calm	Loving	Joyful	Adventurous

Open	Spiritual	Free	Faithful	Generous

What did you learn today?

I AM FEARLESS.

DATE: M   T   W   TH   F   S   S

WEEK # 13   TOTAL HOURS SLEPT:

TONIGHT'S BEDTIME GOAL:

♥ TODAY, I AM GRATEFUL FOR:

🧘 SELF-CARE GOAL(S):

PRAYER REQUEST:

⚔ PERSONAL AFFIRMATION:

🔋 VITAMINS, SUPPLEMENTS & MEDICATIONS

....

....

....

🖊 HEALTH SYMPTOMS

....

....

....

HOW DO I FEEL?(A.M.) ☺ ☹ 😐   HOW DO I FEEL?(P.M.) ☺ ☹ 😐

ENERGY LEVEL ① ② ③ ④ ⑤   ENERGY LEVEL ① ② ③ ④ ⑤

☀ SUN & FRESH AIR ....   🖥 SCREEN TIME ....

ON A CLEANSE? Y / N   ALCOHOL 🍷 🍷 🍷 🍷 🍷

TODAY'S DIET:

✕ FOOD LOG ✕

BREAKFAST	LUNCH	DINNER	SNACK

WATER INTAKE 🌢🌢🌢🌢🌢🌢🌢🌢 TOTAL CALORIES:

⬤━⬤ EXERCISE LOG ⬤━⬤

(OPTIONAL) WEIGHT:				START TIME	END TIME
STRETCH					

WEIGHT TRAINING	WEIGHT	SETS	REPS	START TIME	END TIME

CARDIO	START TIME	END TIME

Circle how you feel today or write your own: ....

Kind   Connected   Clear   Playful   Simple   Abundant

Purposeful   Calm   Loving   Joyful   Adventurous

Open   Spiritual   Free   Faithful   Generous

What did you learn today?

I AM WORTHY.

DATE: M   T   W   TH   F   S   S

WEEK # 13   TOTAL HOURS SLEPT:

TONIGHT'S BEDTIME GOAL:

♥ TODAY, I AM GRATEFUL FOR:

🧘 SELF-CARE GOAL(S):

PRAYER REQUEST:

⚔ PERSONAL AFFIRMATION:

🔋 VITAMINS, SUPPLEMENTS & MEDICATIONS

....

....

....   🌡 HEALTH SYMPTOMS

....

....

....

HOW DO I FEEL?(A.M.) ☺ ☹ 😐   HOW DO I FEEL?(P.M.) ☺ ☹ 😐

ENERGY LEVEL ❶ ❷ ❸ ❹ ❺   ENERGY LEVEL ❶ ❷ ❸ ❹ ❺

🌅 SUN & FRESH AIR ....   🖥 SCREEN TIME ....

ON A CLEANSE?   Y / N   ALCOHOL 🍷 🍷 🍷 🍷 🍷 🍷

TODAY'S DIET:

✖ FOOD LOG ✖

BREAKFAST	LUNCH	DINNER	SNACK

WATER INTAKE 🌢🌢🌢🌢🌢🌢🌢🌢 TOTAL CALORIES:

◁—◉ EXERCISE LOG ◉—▷

(OPTIONAL) WEIGHT:				START TIME	END TIME
STRETCH 🧘					

WEIGHT TRAINING 🏋	WEIGHT	SETS	REPS	START TIME	END TIME

CARDIO 🏃		START TIME	END TIME

Circle how you feel today or write your own: ....

Kind   Connected   Clear   Playful   Simple   Abundant

Purposeful   Calm   Loving   Joyful   Adventurous

Open   Spiritual   Free   Faithful   Generous

What did you learn today?

I AM POWERFUL.

DATE:		M	T	W	TH	F	S	S

WEEK # 13   TOTAL HOURS SLEPT:

TONIGHT'S BEDTIME GOAL:

♥ TODAY, I AM GRATEFUL FOR:

🧘 SELF-CARE GOAL(S):

PRAYER REQUEST:

⚔ PERSONAL AFFIRMATION:

🔋 VITAMINS, SUPPLEMENTS & MEDICATIONS

....
....
....   🌡 HEALTH SYMPTOMS
....
....
....

HOW DO I FEEL?(A.M.) ☺ ☹ 😐   HOW DO I FEEL?(P.M.) ☺ ☹ 😐

ENERGY LEVEL ❶ ❷ ❸ ❹ ❺   ENERGY LEVEL ❶ ❷ ❸ ❹ ❺

☀ SUN & FRESH AIR ....   💻 SCREEN TIME ....

ON A CLEANSE? Y / N   ALCOHOL 🍷 🍷 🍷 🍷 🍷

TODAY'S DIET:

✗ FOOD LOG ✗

BREAKFAST	LUNCH	DINNER	SNACK

WATER INTAKE 🔹🔹🔹🔹🔹🔹🔹🔹 TOTAL CALORIES:

◐—◗ EXERCISE LOG ◐—◗					

(OPTIONAL) WEIGHT:				START TIME	END TIME
STRETCH					
WEIGHT TRAINING	WEIGHT	SETS	REPS	START TIME	END TIME
CARDIO				START TIME	END TIME

Circle how you feel today or write your own: ....

Kind	Connected	Clear	Playful	Simple	Abundant
Purposeful	Calm	Loving	Joyful		Adventurous
Open	Spiritual	Free	Faithful		Generous

What did you learn today?

I AM THANKFUL

DATE: M   T   W   TH   F   S   S

WEEK # 13   TOTAL HOURS SLEPT:

TONIGHT'S BEDTIME GOAL:

♥ TODAY, I AM GRATEFUL FOR:

🧘 SELF-CARE GOAL(S):

PRAYER REQUEST:

⚔ PERSONAL AFFIRMATION:

🔋 VITAMINS, SUPPLEMENTS & MEDICATIONS

....

....

....   🖊 HEALTH SYMPTOMS

....

....

....

HOW DO I FEEL?(A.M.) ☺ ☹ 😐   HOW DO I FEEL?(P.M.) ☺ ☹ 😐

ENERGY LEVEL ❶ ❷ ❸ ❹ ❺   ENERGY LEVEL ❶ ❷ ❸ ❹ ❺

☀ SUN & FRESH AIR ....   📱 SCREEN TIME ....

ON A CLEANSE? Y / N   ALCOHOL 🍷 🍷 🍷 🍷 🍷 🍷

TODAY'S DIET:

✕ FOOD LOG ✕

BREAKFAST	LUNCH	DINNER	SNACK

WATER INTAKE 🌢🌢🌢🌢🌢🌢🌢🌢 TOTAL CALORIES:

⊪—⊪ EXERCISE LOG ⊪—⊪					

(OPTIONAL) WEIGHT:				START TIME	END TIME
STRETCH					
WEIGHT TRAINING	WEIGHT	SETS	REPS	START TIME	END TIME

CARDIO		START TIME	END TIME

Circle how you feel today or write your own: ....

Kind   Connected   Clear   Playful   Simple   Abundant

Purposeful   Calm   Loving   Joyful   Adventurous

Open   Spiritual   Free   Faithful   Generous

What did you learn today?

DATE: M   T   W   TH   F   S   S

WEEK # 13   TOTAL HOURS SLEPT:

TONIGHT'S BEDTIME GOAL:

♥ TODAY, I AM GRATEFUL FOR:

🧘 SELF-CARE GOAL(S):

PRAYER REQUEST:

✗ PERSONAL AFFIRMATION:

🔋 VITAMINS, SUPPLEMENTS & MEDICATIONS

....

....

....   🌡 HEALTH SYMPTOMS

....

....

....

HOW DO I FEEL?(A.M.) ☺ ☹ 😐   HOW DO I FEEL?(P.M.) ☺ ☹ 😐

ENERGY LEVEL ❶ ❷ ❸ ❹ ❺   ENERGY LEVEL ❶ ❷ ❸ ❹ ❺

☀ SUN & FRESH AIR ....   📱 SCREEN TIME ....

ON A CLEANSE? Y / N   ALCOHOL 🍷 🍷 🍷 🍷 🍷

TODAY'S DIET:

✗ FOOD LOG ✗

BREAKFAST	LUNCH	DINNER	SNACK

WATER INTAKE 🌢🌢🌢🌢🌢🌢🌢🌢 TOTAL CALORIES:

I AM BLESSED.

⫸═⫷ EXERCISE LOG ⫸═⫷					

(OPTIONAL) WEIGHT:				START TIME	END TIME
STRETCH 🧘					
WEIGHT TRAINING 🏋	WEIGHT	SETS	REPS	START TIME	END TIME
CARDIO 🚶				START TIME	END TIME

Circle how you feel today or write your own:...

Kind	Connected	Clear	Playful	Simple	Abundant

Purposeful   Calm   Loving   Joyful   Adventurous

Open   Spiritual   Free   Faithful   Generous

What did you learn today?

I AM BRAVE!

DATE:		M	T	W	TH	F	S	S

WEEK # 13   TOTAL HOURS SLEPT:

TONIGHT'S BEDTIME GOAL:

♥ TODAY, I AM GRATEFUL FOR:

🧘 SELF-CARE GOAL(S):

PRAYER REQUEST:

⚔ PERSONAL AFFIRMATION:

⚡ VITAMINS, SUPPLEMENTS & MEDICATIONS

....

....

....   🖊 HEALTH SYMPTOMS

....

....

....

HOW DO I FEEL?(A.M.) ☺ ☹ 😐   HOW DO I FEEL?(P.M.) ☺ ☹ 😐

ENERGY LEVEL ① ② ③ ④ ⑤   ENERGY LEVEL ① ② ③ ④ ⑤

☀ SUN & FRESH AIR ....   💻 SCREEN TIME ....

ON A CLEANSE? Y / N   ALCOHOL 🍷 🍷 🍷 🍷 🍷

TODAY'S DIET:

✖ FOOD LOG ✖

BREAKFAST	LUNCH	DINNER	SNACK

WATER INTAKE 🌢🌢🌢🌢🌢🌢🌢🌢 TOTAL CALORIES:

⫸━⫷ EXERCISE LOG ⫸━⫷					

(OPTIONAL) WEIGHT:				START TIME	END TIME
STRETCH 🧘					

WEIGHT TRAINING 🏋	WEIGHT	SETS	REPS	START TIME	END TIME

CARDIO 🏃	START TIME	END TIME

Circle how you feel today or write your own: ....

Kind	Connected	Clear	Playful	Simple	Abundant
Purposeful	Calm	Loving	Joyful		Adventurous
Open	Spiritual	Free	Faithful		Generous

What did you learn today?

_____

_____

_____

_____

_____

_____

_____

_____

_____

_____

_____

_____

_____

WELLNESS APPOINTMENTS: _____

_____

_____

NEEDS IMPROVEMENT: _____

_____

_____

INSIGHTS & LESSONS: _____

_____

_____

SUCCESSES & WINS: _____

_____

_____

_____

WEEKLY CHECK-IN

END DATE:

(optional) Measurements

Waist: Chest:

Thighs: Hips:

Upper Arms: Calves:

What was your biggest accomplishment in the past 90 days?

What did you discover about yourself using this wellness journal?

CONGRATULATIONS! You finished the journey, how do you feel?

Kind	Connected	Clear	Playful	Simple	Abundant
Purposeful	Calm	Loving	Joyful	Adventurous
Open	Spiritual	Free	Faithful	Generous

Made in the USA
Columbia, SC
27 November 2023

27209653R00122